DISCOVER
THE DOCTOR
Within

J.E. BLOCK, M.D. F.A.C.P.

BLOCKHAUS PUBLISHING
TULSA, OK

DISCOVER THE DOCTOR WITHIN
IT'S NOT HOW OLD YOU ARE,
BUT HOW YOU ARE WHEN YOU'RE OLD.

J. E. BLOCK, MD, F.A.C.P.

The opinions in this book are strictly those of the author and not necessarily those of any professional group. As a physician I do give medical advice, but on a specific individual basis. Therefore, nothing in this book should be construed as my medical opinion to the reader.

Copyright 2011, J. E. Block, MD
ISBN: 978-1-42765261-4
Library of Congress Control Number

DEDICATION

This book is dedicated to you my patients for the inspiration. To my parents for the intellect. And most of all, to my wife, Brunhilde, and our eight children, fifteen grandchildren, and three great-grandchildren for their sacrifices to allow me to be the doctor I am today.

Previous Books

Electrocardiographic Interpretations

Cardiac Rehabilitation Techniques

*A Horse and Buggy Doctor Caught
in the Twenty-First Century*

Secrets to a Longer and Better Life

If you would like to order another or
several of *Discover the Doctor Within,*
write to
P.O. Box 35422
Tulsa, Oklahoma 74153
or
Visit my website
docblock.com

THE HIPPOCRATIC OATH

I swear by Apollo the physician, by Aesculapius, Hygeia, and Panacea, and I take to witness all the gods, all the goddesses, to keep according to my ability and my judgment the following oath:

To consider dear to me as my parents him who taught me this art; to live in common with him and if necessary to share my goods with him; to look upon his children as my own brothers, to teach them this art if they so desire without fee or written promise; to impart to my sons and the sons of the master who taught me and the disciples who have enrolled themselves and have agreed to the rules of the profession, but to these alone, the precepts and the instruction. I will prescribe regimen for the good of my patients according to my ability and my judgment and never do harm to anyone. To please no one will I prescribe a deadly drug, nor give advice which may cause his death. Nor will I give a woman a pessary to procure abortion. But I will preserve the purity of my life and my art. I will not cut for stone, even for patients in whom the disease is manifest; I will leave this operation to be performed by practitioners (specialists in this art). In every house where I come I will enter only for the good of my patients, keeping myself far from all intentional ill-doing and all seduction, and especially from the pleasures of love with women or with men, be they free or slaves. All that may come to my knowledge in the exercise of my profession or in daily commerce with men, which ought not to be spread abroad, I will keep secret and never reveal. If I keep this oath faithfully may I enjoy my life and practice my art, respected by all men and in all times; but if I swerve from it or violate it, may the reverse be my lot.

TABLE OF CONTENTS

5. Forever Young

6. Materia Medical

INTRODUCTION

O ur toxic environment and modern lifestyle are killing us from the inside out. Degenerative and near-epidemic diseases such as obesity, arthritis, arteriosclerosis, Alzheimer's, osteoporosis, premature aging, and iatrogenic (caused by the healer) disease have tragically become part of every American family. Yet as technology advances, the wisdom of the ages proves that it was better to *prevent* than to treat disease.

Two doctors, three opinions are given, but the opinion that is the most important is **YOURS**, the patient. It is not the physician who will suffer the most if good therapies go on getting it wrong, an adverse drug reaction occurs, or the operation was a success, but the patient died, but you and your family should be in charge of your health both preventively and therapeutically! A healing relationship with your physician is important, and teamwork is key, but it should be you as the patient who is responsible for the path to take. The doctor is the knowledgeable coach or advisor, perhaps a family member, too, could be the team manager, but there is no doubt that if you are in your right mind, the decision of care should be yours! It is incumbent for you to be as knowledgeable as possible on the medical problem at hand. Information from the Internet, perhaps starting at Wikipedia, then a noncommercial website, such as WebMD, should be considered. Speaking to other patients with a similar problem, as well as reading magazine articles or books can give a good working knowledge on your medical issue. Even getting another professional opinion from a physician who is not in cahoots with your original doc is a good idea.

Too often primary care physicians function as gate-keepers; they may open the floodgates and let the patient drown in too many medical procedures and medicines. Fragmentation in medical care also is rampant today. The patient who decides what organ or area their problem lies in sees that specialist. Therefore, there is a cardiologist for their heart, a pulmonologist for their lungs, a nephrologist for their kidneys, a hematologist for their blood, and a "Big Toe doctor" for their gout. That leaves us with no one to take care of the whole person; moreover, the left hand doesn't know what the right hand is doing. The gastroenterologist does not effectively communicate with the neurologist. If your primary care doctor does not function as a knowledgeable clinical coordinator, then that responsibility by default falls to you. As I try to set forth in this book, it is not how old a person is that counts, but how they feel and function when they are old. Medicine and certainly not this book alone have all the answers, but with your significant participation you will enable yourself to age gracefully and to live a full and abundant life. It is imperative, then, to DISCOVER THE DOCTOR WITHIN!

1

A Prelude to Health

Throughout history, mankind has continually searched for the secret to a long and healthy life. Today medical science has provided us with a wealth of information on how to achieve this goal. Yet we also must remember the wisdom that it is far better to *prevent* disease than it is to *cure* it—and we must not forsake this innate sense that has kept mankind alive and thriving for thousands of years.

Good Medicine

So where does a long and healthy life begin? It starts with a pure internal and external environment. Our individual genetic endowments ultimately produce, as God intended, an integrally happy human being, assuming appropriate pre- and postnatal care is provided. As we grow, we must learn how to communicate internally by listening to our bodies, and externally by listening to our environment.

In other words, there is much more to a healthy life than simply avoiding the medical establishment with its knives, poisons, and burns (especially from radiation). A connection to a higher power, sincere companionship, and a vital relationship with one's significant other are key ingredients in life's recipe for health. Furthermore, volunteering to help others, not taking ourselves too seriously, and knowing life is to be enjoyed, not endured, contribute to an abundant life. Health, therefore, encompasses much more than an absence of illness.

This concept is often lost on the medical community. The historian and surgeon Sherwin B. Newland stated that medical advances in the past 2,500 years have come not from a steady continuum of progress, but from quantum leaps in knowledge and practice, usually by those who thought "out of the box." Why then, despite the tremendous advances we have made scientifically, are doctors still, as a profession, third-rate physicians practicing fourth-rate medicine? It is not, I suggest, because of a pervasive lack of knowledge, but because of the traditional medical mind-set. Most physicians are blinded to many scientific studies that should confirm rather than contradict medical theory. This blindness might be acceptable in other academic endeavors, but medicine is an art based on scientific principles. Thus, research should verify hypotheses, confirm theories, and document presumed truths. But because of our cultural biases and emotional prejudices, the evolution of medicine has been stuck in a quagmire of half-truths and pseudo-facts that sometimes borders on junk science. What we surmise as medical fact today may well be false tomorrow. Over the past fifty years as a physician I have seen this repeatedly. Medical knowledge is doubling every five years, yet we live in a forest of medical information without knowing the true nature of the trees.

The relationship of estrogen and breast cancer is an example of this uncomfortable evolution. Prior to 1950 no relationship had been established. In the late sixties, some literature began to suggest that giving estrogen to a woman post-menopause *might* cause cancer. In the eighties there was proof that it actually *did* cause cancer. By the early nineties, however, it was discovered that estrogen did not cause cancer of the breast, but would accelerate its growth in women who *already had* the cancer. In 2011, bioidentical estrogen is given to women with breast cancer by either truly gifted physicians or quacks. What, then, is a person to believe?

While scientific breakthroughs in medicine uncover pieces of the puzzle, most often still more research is needed to confirm the data and fit the pieces together. Medical knowledge is always in a state of flux. However, we live in today's world based on yesterday's facts, not tomorrow's assumptions. Thus, thousands of years of human experience should not be dismissed in favor of so-called modern scientific research. Both must contribute to understanding health, and in the future the true relationship of hormones and cancer will be discovered.

The development of our medical perspective on tobacco in health demonstrates this understanding of the connection between "common sense" experience and scientific medical research.

We have known intuitively for over two hundred years that smoking is bad for us. Still, tobacco companies have tried to seduce us into thinking that it was not harmful. For instance, according to a 1951 advertisement in *LIFE* magazine, most doctors advised smoking for relaxation, with over 85 percent of doctors smoking themselves (See Figure I-1 on page 20). Today more than 85 percent of doctors do not smoke, and none advise it. However, it was not until 1964 that the Surgeon General acknowledged that, based on scientific studies, smoking causes illnesses, and only now are the tobacco companies successfully being sued for injury although the harmfulness of smoking is a medical truth that will never change, although other nicotine delivery systems such as the E-cigarette, the vaporizer, or the best, non-tobacco-derived nicotine, are another story.

Do we need a hundred double-blind studies costing billions of dollars to prove what your grandmother knew through common sense? The answer to this is both yes and no. At times, what we have believed to be true for a hundred years suddenly turns out to be false. For example, malaria is not caused by breathing bad air, as "common sense" had dictated, but, as Dr. Walter Reed proved, by the bite of an

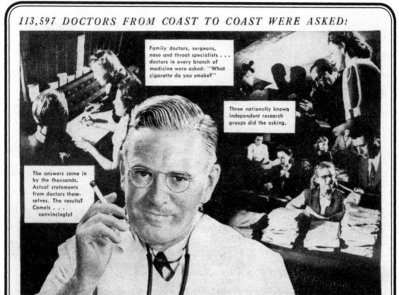

113,597 DOCTORS FROM COAST TO COAST WERE ASKED!

According to this recent Nationwide survey:

R. J. Reynolds Tobacco Co., Winston-Salem, N. C.

MORE DOCTORS SMOKE CAMELS THAN ANY OTHER CIGARETTE!

This is no casual claim. It's an actual fact. Based on the statements of doctors themselves to three nationally known independent research organizations.

THE QUESTION was very simple. One that you . . . any smoker . . . might ask a doctor: "What cigarette do you smoke, Doctor?"

After all, doctors are human too. Like you, they smoke for pleasure. Their taste, like yours, enjoys the pleasing flavor of costlier tobaccos. Their throats too appreciate a cool mildness.

And more doctors named Camels than any other cigarette!

If you are a Camel smoker, this preference for Camels among physicians and surgeons will not surprise you. But

if you are not now smoking Camels, try them. Compare them in your "T-Zone."

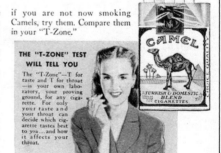

THE "T-ZONE" TEST WILL TELL YOU

The "T-Zone"—T for taste and T for throat —is your own laboratory, your proving ground, for any cigarette. For only your taste and your throat can decide which cigarette tastes best to you . . . and how it affects your throat.

CAMEL — COSTLIER TOBACCOS

Figure I-1

infected mosquito. This kind of discovery is now popularized as *evidence-based medicine*. It reminds us to have open minds, but it still does not prove that if it is not taught in medical school and if it is not published in several peer review medical journals, it is not so.

Evidence-based medicine as noted in the introduction must be understood in its current context: Today most of us realize that what is published is either economically driven by pharmaceutical companies or is dictated by medical politics. It is now law that if a study disproves a pharmacologic intervention, it still has to be published despite the negative press for the drug company. But this is certainly not acknowledged in well-read scientific journals. Despite what mainstream medicine supports, treatments that have not been proven "scientifically" are not necessarily *disproved* and can be useful in medical practice.

In this new millennium we should strive to increase the quality as well as the quantity of our lives. What good is a long life if one does not live well? At any age, we should be physically and mentally as young as possible. It is not important how old we are, but rather how we are when we are old. An old German saying states, "A healthy person has many desires; the sick individual has but one—to be healthy."

Having a healthy life takes lots of work, good genes, faith, and a pinch of luck. Many of us believe that, like a broken piece of machinery, our bodies can be fixed as good as new through medicine or surgery. This is not so if we become injured or ill! With every illness, every disease, every trauma, a small but permanent disability remains. Thus, we must learn how to take better care of ourselves today so there will be minimal disability tomorrow. How can we bring this to fruition in our own lives? Should we believe our doctor, the new health magazine, Grandma, or ourselves? Ultimately, being informed and assertive in our health care will give us the best chance for a healthier future. The rest of this book will show you how you can do this—in your own life—to be your own doctor.

An Ounce of Prevention

Ben Franklin had it right: It is certainly better to prevent than to treat disease. The former is referred to as "prophylactic" or "preventive" medicine, and the latter is "crisis medicine." Most allopathic physicians (MDs and DOs) practice crisis medicine, such as treating acute organ damage (e.g., heart attack), infection (e.g., appendicitis), or trauma (e.g., a fractured bone). The concept that many illnesses are caused by our modern way of life, as opposed to that of our ancestors, is not wrong. Illnesses that occur because of our changing environment are referred to as degenerative diseases. They include arthritis, arteriosclerosis, Alzheimer's disease, chronic fatigue syndrome, poor vision, and even aging itself.

Yes, aging, at least prematurely, is considered an actual disease by some. Genetically, we should be destined to live 120 to 140 years; but because of our environment, a decrease in glandular secretion (hormones), and faulty genes (those that decrease immunity or produce organ abnormalities), we do not live to our full life expectancy. The Genome Project has proven that our genes are indeed malleable. One's life can vary depending on which gene is stimulated and which is suppressed by the environment. With the advent of genetic engineering, we can actually begin life as perfect humans. Prenatal care can ensure that the untainted embryo is programmed to be a healthy baby, and subsequently, a wholesome, mature person. Then, a combination of crisis intervention and prevention should allow us not only to reach our full quality but quantity of life, to stay in our prime for at least a century.

Never Too Old

All that is needed for the preservation of a species is for an organism to survive for enough time to produce and nurture offspring long enough for them to survive on their own. In the case of humans, this occurs when the mother has nourished, protected, and taught her child how to make it alone in the hostile world. The father often helps to foster, protect, and teach, although his primary biological purpose is to fertilize the egg. Subsequently, after producing two or more offspring, the parents are no longer needed for the maintenance of the species. After a given time, first the ovaries, then other glandular secretions gradually decrease in the woman. The male often maintains some testicular secretion (testosterone), but this too, wanes as he ages.

Thanks to research, we can now replace or enhance almost all of these glandular secretions, or hormones. Thus, we do not have to succumb to the unnatural state of diminishing endocrine function and disability. As a result, human parents, grandparents, and other adults work with children not only until they grow up, but they continue the education, protection, and nourishment until the offspring are fully integrated into society. It is a delight to be a parent, a bigger joy to be a grandparent, and a jubilation to be a great-grandparent, as I am. Today, being a great-great-grandparent is the exception; tomorrow it will be the rule. Even after their reproductive years are over, people can continue to contribute to society in many beneficial ways. Thus, the endeavors of people from maturity to death a century later will improve technical science, cultivate cultural discoveries, and enhance the lives of humankind, both present and future. Although society has generally put older folks out to pasture, this is also changing. Older people are useful not just as greeters in Walmart, but are back in their previous technical jobs. In the future, we will not be forced to retire just because of age, our community, and our current income tax structure. We will be physically, mentally, and economically productive for as long as we desire and the Lord has planned.

The World Has Changed

A balanced union of mind, body, and spirit will allow human beings to achieve their full destiny. The spirit, be it the holy or natural life force, must be present for us to exist. I do believe in a Divine Creator, but as a scientist, I also believe in evolution—not the classic Darwinian model, but a form of long-term incremental development "guided by a higher power." Mankind has evolved over the last four hundred thousand years. Since research has disclosed that it takes at least twenty thousand years to produce a new species, we are still, metabolically, Paleolithic (cavemen). As hunter-gatherers, our ancestors could, perhaps, have survived to 120 years if not for crisis illnesses and dangerous environmental conditions like inadequate food, shelter, and sanitation, as well as the presence of enemies. While our ability to treat and control these circumstances has improved, other hazards have evolved with modern society.

High-density carbohydrates such as sugar, starches, and alcohol are products of humanity's mental rather than physical evolution. Grains did not exist as a reliable food source until the last twelve thousand years. The great majority of us are still not genetically adapted to metabolizing these, and grains will eventually turn out to be a curse rather than a blessing to mankind. Yes, they do feed the masses, but in the land of plenty they cause premature disability and *death*. To add insult to injury, the minerals we need to stay at our metabolic best have diminished through the depletion of our soil over the centuries. Magnesium, for example, is a plant/animal mineral and an essential component of chlorophyll, a necessary catalyst for plant growth. Our magnesium intake is only a fraction of what it should be; in fact, almost 40 percent of us are magnesium-deficient by the time we reach the ripe old age of twenty! The replacement of this important mineral is now known to "cure" hypertension, high cholesterol, diabetes, osteoporosis, muscle cramps, arthritis, and heart disease. Similarly, minerals such as zinc, copper, iron, calcium, chromium, and selenium were abundant in the diet of our hunter-gatherer ancestors, but they are not today. To make matters worse, water has been "purified" to such an extent that electrons, trace minerals, and rare minerals that were naturally included are now excluded from its live or flowing form and toxins such as chlorine and fluoride are added.

If the deprivation of minerals is not enough to cause our modern-day diseases, the presence of poisons in our environment destroys our current biochemistry. These can include pesticides in our food, hydrocarbons in our dry-cleaned clothes, radiation and electromagnetic waves to which we are exposed, noxious chemicals we apply to our bodies, and pollutants in the air. Furthermore, we now insulate our houses for better energy conservation than we did fifty years ago that we have tripled the concentration of some of these harmful compounds to which we are exposed.

FAITH AS A HEALER

Over twelve hundred research studies and reports indicate that spirituality and religion are extremely important determinants to health. In his book, *A Century of Research Reviewed*, Harold Koenig, MD, includes an extensive discussion of the healing power of faith. For instance, in double-blind studies, bypass surgery patients who had no idea they were being prayed for did much better than a similar group for which there were no prayers. The prayers came from various denominations hundreds of miles away.

The healing power of faith is based not only on the mysterious, but also on overlooked psychological principles. The physical and spiritual support of a temple, church, or mosque, for example, can help relieve a patient's sense of isolation and a consuming obsession with his or her problems, thereby improving mental health and adaptation to disability. This, in turn, plays a large role in stress relief. Helping others to enrich their lives can help mentally and biophysically through the production of healthy internal secretions. In this context of faith and healing, we know that the cytokines, natural inflammatory chemicals involved in damage to our tissues, are significantly lower in folks who attended religious services compared to those who did not.

The lifestyle or behavior codes of many systems of faith also encourage good health. Negative health behaviors such as smoking and alcohol consumption are often tempered or prohibited. Moderation in personal and professional affairs, as well as in duty and pleasure, is widely advocated. Even for the generally healthy, religious activities are associated with a six- to ten-year longer survival than those who practice no religion, according to a study by Dr. D. Oman in the *American Journal of Public Health*. Considering its spiritual, psychological, scientific, and commonsensical influence, it is no wonder that organized religion has grown by 10 percent annually in America.

THE WAVES OF ENERGY

Other bioenergetic systems such as the Chinese meridian concept are used by acupuncturists and in electroconductive analysis. They are frequently documented but poorly understood in terms of anatomy and biochemistry. However, they are medically useful in spite of our incomplete understanding. We know that, depending on the wavelengths, energy is transmitted from the invisible to the visible.

The Bible commands, "Let there be light," but we do not get enough, nor the right kind. For eons human beings bathed in light by day and hid in darkness by night. Civilization, however, has changed all this. We use artificial light at night and are deprived of natural light during the day. The artificial light used in our homes, schools, and workplaces is not full-spectrum and is therefore not nearly as good for our bodies as the sunlight we naturally need. Even being washed by sunlight through a window is not as healthy as being outdoors, because glass filters out some of its robust vitality. It is well known that SAD (Seasonal Affective Disorder) is caused by not getting enough outside light in the fall and winter. Moreover, it has been found that the use of full-spectrum light during the day is a successful treatment for some depressive disorders. Sleep disorders, daytime fatigue, and poor concentration are also improved by getting full-spectrum light for one hour in the morning. Sleeping in a very dark, quiet room helps, as well.

Certain spectrums of light (colors) change neuropeptides in the brain that not only elevate one's mood, but also heal. Various colors can be used to treat maladies such as headaches, gastrointestinal problems, and congestion. Light exerts some of its effects through regulating the hormone melatonin, produced in the pituitary gland. Melatonin helps us harmonize with changes in the environment, especially in daily and seasonal transitions of our sun.

Not Enough Sleep

True insomnia includes difficulty falling asleep, getting up in the middle of the night and not easily falling back to sleep, or getting up extremely early in the morning. However, insomnia can also be illusory. A recent Oxford study in *The Journal of Sleep* indicated that some people do not have true insomnia, but erroneously think they do. This is pseudo-insomnia, which is related to the overestimation of the time between closing the eyes until sleep, an underestimation of total sleep time, and a longer cognitive arousal period (reporting having been awake just before they were awakened). These give a distorted perception of sleep and the impression of insomnia where there may actually be none.

In a sleep laboratory—where there is monitoring of the brain waves—movement, temperature, and respiratory rate disclosed a mismatch between perception and reality. The proof of the pudding is in the eating. If one perceives they have poor sleep, they will feel it, and a vicious negative cycle ensues. The increased anxiety and worry of not getting a good night's sleep will actually cause a poor night's sleep!

How long should a person really sleep each night? Published articles indicate that the more a person sleeps, the more likely it is that they will lose weight. Another study published in *The Journal of Sleep* from Japan, showed those who slept between 6.5 and 7.5 hours on weekdays had the best survival rates. But the mortality risk of those who slept *more than* 7.5 hours was greater than those who slept 6.5!

Those who reported sleeping nine hours a night had a greater mortality risk than those who slept one hour less. The *Nurses Health Study* and *Cancer Prevention Study* reached a very similar conclusion. These studies involved over a quarter of a million people.

Is a nap helpful? I believe so, despite a study in Israel several years ago that concluded that following a nap there was a slightly higher increase in having a cardiovascular event (just like "normally" occurs when one gets up from their night's sleep in the morning). If one were to take a nap, the best time would be to capitalize on the post-lunch dip of core body temperature with an increased likelihood of easy sleep initiation. In other words, if you do want to take a nap, you will likely be able to fall asleep easier right after lunch.

Microwaves and Microbrains

Microwave radiation increases free radical destruction of our tissue. Cell phones are one major source for microwave damage. In particular, the electromagnetic radiation emitted by cell phones penetrates the adjacent neural tissue. The larger the brain is relative to the body, the greater the risk. This is why some researchers who study cell phone damage to humans advise that children, who have a larger brain/body ratio than adults, should not use them. Recently, twenty-one studies on cell phone radiation were reviewed. None of them demonstrated that cell phone radiation is safe. The risks range from miniscule to more destruction of brain tissue and an increase incidence of tumors. To be truthful, the research was poorly controlled, based on people remembering the details about their cell phone use. Also, older studies on rats were reviewed by the FDA prior to the release of cell phones and showed there was "no significant damage to the DNA." However, we are not rats and there may be a genetic predisposition to neurologic dysfunction and to cancer in some of us. But, to date, there is no easy way in determining who of us have this tendency, and so we all should be cautious with our cell phone use.

Free radicals generated by microwaves can be neutralized by our natural antioxidant system, especially by superoxide dismutase and glutathione peroxidase. These can be augmented by gingko biloba, resveratrol, and quercitin (found in fresh fruits). The farther the source of the microwave is away from the brain, the smaller the problem. However, an earpiece attachment is still dangerous in that the microwaves are transmitted around the wire. An iron bead in the middle of the wire can diminish much of the damaging effect of this radiation. Even those devices that aren't connected by wire, such as bluetooth, produce some microwave radiation.

So, what is a person to do? Common sense dictates that the less time spent with the instrument next to your head, the better. Another solution is a speakerphone. Even better, use a blue *tube* device, which, much like a stethoscope, transmits sound from a small amplifier twelve inches from the brain through a small conduit to the ear.

As to whether or not cell phones cause brain cancer and Alzheimer's disease, no one knows for sure, but the great experiment on millions of people is ongoing and the next decade will show if there indeed is a problem. I would prefer not to be exposed to much microradiation and ten years from now find that it was benign, than expose myself and subsequently find I have the beginning of Alzheimer's or, worse, a brain tumor!

Microwave ovens are a different case since their wave size is quite large and less likely to escape the blocking mesh of the oven door.

Captain of the Team

Most physicians go into medicine for the proper humanitarian reasons, to help people. However, many of us emerge from medical training with a different spin on life. Most doctors end up overly self-interested, looking for both ego and economic fulfillment. Some retain their calling and remain compassionate healers. Good doctors are born, not made. Sure, we need medical scientists, but they should stay in research, teach some, and practice little or none. How, then, does a patient find a physician who thinks with his mind and feels with his heart? We need someone who is kind, who has time to listen, and who is seasoned, not too young nor too old. He or she should be accessible and, most importantly, understand the mind-body interaction. He or she should be open-minded enough to respect our opinions on both conventional and alternative therapies. I am referring to a primary care doctor who, if he is good, knows what he knows and, more significantly, knows what he does not know. And if he does not know something, he will find someone for us who does! If there are 2 doctors there are 3 opinions and the most important opinion comes from the doctor within!

Frugal doctors sometimes achieve more by doing and spending less. Prevention always trumps medication, and natural medicine may be better than drugs and procedures that are expensive, dangerous, and perhaps, not even proven to be effective. The 9,000 patient *NAVIGATOR* study, completed in 2009, found the antihypertensive drug Diovan (Valsatan) kept 14 percent of patients who were diabetes-prone from developing the disease. It did *not*, however, prevent any of the cardiovascular events that make diabetes so devastating.

The *ASTRAL* study of almost 1,000 patients, finished in 2010, showed that patients with high blood pressure from narrowed arteries in their kidneys, and who received stents, did *not* experience lower blood pressure. They *did*, however, experience more unfavorable side effects—including death!

Frequently, there is a gap between what we expect as a patient and what we receive. In these days of managed care, we are often assigned a doctor rather than allowed to choose one. If you are medically knowledgeable, (and after reading this book you should be more so!), I recommend interviewing your prospective physician. Offer to pay for his or her time. In addition to the usual questions about fees and insurance coverage, ask how he or she feels about disease prevention, nutrition, and natural remedies. *You* should be the captain of your medical team (the doctor within) and your physician the coach. Make sure the staff is courteous, helpful, and treats you like an individual, not like another poor patient in need of medical help.

The Internet, the Yellow Pages, county medical society secretaries, and hospitals have lists of primary care physicians (PCPs). They are referenced as family medicine practitioners, general internists, and gynecologists. Also, any physician, regardless of specialty, can be holistic and have the proper philosophy to take care of your entire person. Too often PCPs function as gate keepers; they may open the floodgates and let the patient drown in too many medical procedures and medicines. The government, the AMA, Medicare, and Medicaid are going to push for medical unification so the fragmentation of medical care will disappear. Fragmentation in medical care is rampant today. The patient who decides what organ or area their problem lies in sees that specialist. Therefore, there is a cardiologist for their heart, a pulmonologist for their lungs, a nephrologist for their kidneys, a hematologist for their blood, and a "Big Toe doctor" for their gout. That leaves us with no one to take care of the whole person; moreover, the left hand doesn't know what the right hand is doing. The gastroenterologist does not effectively communicate with the neurologist. The new "Medical Home" now being contrived may bring it together.

A Shift in Medical Thinking

It is not *who* is right, but *what* is right that counts. Alternative medicine is being rediscovered and is slowly shifting the medical paradigm; what used to be considered nonscientific bunk, some physicians now think is the correct method of healing a patient. One of the main reasons physicians are hesitant to use alternative medicine is the lack of scientific proof or explanation of its effectiveness. Conventionally trained allopathic physicians evaluate alternative medicine through the biomechanical model and not through the general systems theory, which is more plausible to the variations of the human organism. Therefore, Chinese, Ayurvedic, herbal, and electromagnetic medicine, among others, could, but do not, make sense to most physicians who have had orthodox medical training. There are several important differences between the biomechanical model we learned in medical school and the general systems hypothesis espoused by alternative physicians.

The general systems theory considers quantum physics, which can explain sudden unexpected changes in a person's health. It sees an individual as a total organism rather than a biological machine. The individual strives to maintain stability through homoeostasis, keeping all parts of the body in balance. Thus, a sudden perturbation may be interpreted by the organism as a crisis, in which the body releases potentially noxious chemicals into the bloodstream. The individual then consciously or unconsciously identifies the disturbance and influences it. If, for a simple example, we are cold, we shiver, which produces internal heat. When such attempts to harmonize our internal and external circumstances fail, disease is the result! Another instance: When suffering digestive distress, unless there is significant fluid loss from diarrhea, drugs such as Imodium actually inhibit the person from getting rid of the noxious agent that started the process.

As the changing of the medical paradigm suggests, in the long run, society is frugal; that is, what is not practical has generally been thrown out over the millennia. We have scientifically and philosophically revised medicine again and again. Oriental and other older forms of medicine long ago rid themselves of what did not work; and what has survived succeeds. Although the yin-yang proposition holds little validity to most Western physicians, and the meridian concept with chi may be considered heretical by mainstream doctors, both should have a place in modern medicine. There is a definite need for these types of diagnoses and treatments. In Oriental and Ayurvedic medicine, feeling the pulse, inspecting the tongue, and intuitively sensing what illness the patient has are methods used to diagnose and treat the patient. Some diseases with which modern medicine has a poor track record, such as chronic fatigue syndrome, fibromyalgia, and irritable bowel, may be better diagnosed and treated by these other disciplines.

If a physician cannot account for the underlying explanation of an illness based on the scientific reasoning learned from allopathic medicine, he or she may relegate the patient's problem to the head and not to the body. But if a doctor can otherwise intuit what is going on, he or she is not arbitrarily assigning a cause and can greatly help a patient even though it cannot be documented on the patient's conventional medical chart. A physician is not a magician. Diagnosis and treatment is logic based on relativity, as was claimed by Einstein, rather than on the older, static mechanical physics embraced centuries earlier by Newton. Of course, in today's science, both Newton and Einstein are correct, and the world accepts both. So, why can't this happen with orthodox medicine and unconventional medical concepts? A holistic approach is the only way to treat some disease states. Why not present the best of both worlds to an individual who may need one or the other or, possibly, a combination of these philosophies? The following chapters will expand on this more realistic approach to health. A combination of an open-minded, reasonable physician and a naturopath might well accomplish your health goals.

Our Natural Detoxification

We are exposed to a great number of xenobiotics (foreign compounds) during the course of a lifetime, including a variety of pharmaceuticals and food components. Many of these show little relationship to previously encountered chemicals or metabolites, and yet we are capable of managing environmental exposure by detoxifying them. To accomplish this task, our bodies have evolved a complex organization of detoxification enzymes. But in our toxic world these systems need help. The enzyme systems generally functioned adequately in the past to minimize the potential for damage by xenobiotics. But in our modern civilization, we are being overwhelmed by them. There is an association between impaired detoxification and illness, such as cancer, neurological disease, fibromyalgia, and chronic fatigue/immune dysfunction syndrome. Therefore, an individual's ability to remove toxins from the body plays a role in the cause or flare-up of chronic conditions and new diseases. Natural helpers include the sulfuaranes found in crucifer vegetables such as broccoli and the very best, broccoli sprouts.

Our detoxification systems are highly complex and show a great amount of individual variability. These are extremely responsive to a person's environment, lifestyle, and genetic uniqueness. The liver is the principal organ of detoxification, although all tissue has some ability to metabolize foreign chemicals. The liver is the largest organ, and it is the first body part perfused by chemicals absorbed in the gut. Also there are very high concentrations of most metabolizing enzyme systems relative to other tissues. When food or a drug is taken into the GI tract, it is taken apart in the gut. When it is absorbed into the body, it first enters the hepatic (liver) circulation through the portal vein. Here it is metabolized if possible, before it can go into the rest of the body—and eventually back to the liver again and again. This is the *first pass effect*. When the altered substance is fat-soluble, it is excreted into the bile, then discharged into the intestine, only to be reabsorbed again. This process is repeated many times, hence the term *enterohepatic circulation*.

Factors that affect detoxification are age, individual genetic variation (polymorphism), enterohepatic circulation, nutrition, intestinal flora, gender, and drugs. Other sites of chemical metabolism/excretion include the gastrointestinal tract, the lungs (volatile compounds), the kidneys (water-soluble molecules), and the skin (both lipid- and water-soluble chemicals). These sites at times could have localized toxicity reactions. The detoxification systems are complex. They are divided into three interacting parts or phases, each of which can engage with itself or any of the other two to work in harmony defending our bodies from being acutely or slowly poisoned to death. At times, it is overwhelmed and we rapidly or slowly die.

The three phases of detoxification are termed Phases I, II, and III of Detoxification. Any variation of the activities of these can mean the difference between disease (including drug adversity, cancer, arthritis, cardiovascular disease) and health. To add to the complexity, the phase system is orchestrated by our genetically endowed CYP-450 enzymes that steer or turn them, for better or worse. The initial Phase I metabolism, if possible, makes the ingested chemicals water-soluble to later be eliminated by the kidneys. The subsequent joining of the molecule with a lipid-conjugation occurs in Phase II; it is eliminated through the bile and eventually enters our fecal stream. The newly discovered Phase III gets rid of the offending chemical by importing it into a cell then exporting it out into a storage or excretion system.

Most of the CYP in humans is found in the liver, the main organ involved in drug and toxin removal, but a fair amount is also located in the small intestine. CYP is usually found in the "microsomal" part of the cytoplasm (endoplasmic reticulum).

Metabolic clearance of drugs is not the only function of CYP. Recently it has been found that CYP is involved in vascular autoregulation, particularly in the brain. CYP is involved in the formation of cholesterol, steroids, and arachidonic acid metabolites.

Let's take a closer look at the Three Phases of Detoxification.

Phase I

The Phase I detoxification system, influenced by the cytochrome P450 supergene family of enzymes, is generally the first enzymatic defense against foreign compounds. They are nonsynthetic reactions involving oxidation, reduction, hydrolysis, cyclization, and decyclization. Most of the unwanted and detrimental metabolites and pharmaceuticals are metabolized through the Phase I biotransformation, and it is then excreted. At times reactive molecules, which sometimes may be more toxic than the parent molecule, are produced. If these reactive molecules are not further metabolized by Phase II conjugation, they cause damage to proteins, DNA, and RNA within the cell.

Phase II

Phase II is comprised of conjugation reactions that generally follow Phase I activation, resulting in a xenobiotic that has been transformed into a fat-soluble compound. It can then be excreted through the bile. There are at least four types of conjugation reactions present in the body (glucuronidation, sulfation, glutathione, and amino acid binding). These reactions require cofactors, such as minerals and micronutrients, that must be replenished through dietary sources.

Phase III

Recently antiporter activity has been defined as the Phase III detoxification system. It is an exchanger or counter-transporter on a membrane protein that is involved in active transport of two or more different molecules or ions across a phospholipid membrane in opposite directions. To make it even more complex, there is a secondary active transport; one species of solute moves along its electrochemical gradient, allowing a different species to move against its own electrochemical gradient. This is in contrast to primary active transport, in which all solutes are moved against their concentration gradients, fueled by ATP. The antiporter is an energy-dependent efflux pump, which pumps the chemical in question out of a cell, thereby decreasing the intracellular concentration of xenobiotics. Antiporter activity in the intestine appears to be co-regulated with intestinal Phase I CYP enzymes. One example of the "porter system" is iodide being actively transported into the thyroid.

So if we cannot keep all the poisons out of our bodies, let us at least aid ourselves with helpers such as the natural inducers of the CYP detoxifiers like the crucifers or the best, broccoli sprouts, or even the active ingredients in them, such as DIM or I3C. It will keep us more out of harm's way if we eat and drink to avoid the known toxins in our food and beverages.

Mind over Matter

A good doctor endeavors to help the body repair itself, to awaken the healer within. Thus, we try to approach a patient from several different directions to see what is the most beneficial. This will lead the patient down the correct track toward regained health, preserved wholeness, and a satisfying and abundant life. At any given time the total health of a patient is determined by a series of factors, the most important of which is genetics.

In the past, we have thought of genetics as a fixed determinant. Certainly hair color, skin color, eye color, and height are not easily changed without the help of hair dye, UV light, tinted contact lenses, and growth hormones. We are discovering, however, that much of the genetic code is malleable. At the molecular level we are finding that the internal milieu determines genetic expression. Under certain external conditions the biochemistry of a given piece of the genetic code is stimulated, but under different circumstances another part of the code is activated. For example: If the oncogene p53 is turned on by a methylation transfer, the patient is more likely to get cancer. In other words, the same set of genes will manifest different characteristics in response to the environment. This is referred to as epigenetics.

Therefore, almost ironically, our intimate surroundings determine whether or not we will get an inherited disease like coronary artery disease, breast cancer, prostate cancer, or diabetes. After genetics, the second basic component of the body's structure is the actual building-blocks used to create the individual: Food, drink, and air provide the molecules of which we are composed. Certainly, if one gives the body faulty building materials or fills it with toxins that interfere with its ideal structure, the body will become weakened and vulnerable. The same is true for improper fuel (our food): Not only will our bodies not run properly, but the machine can be damaged for future operation.

Our cells are given specific instructions by certain chemicals or neuropeptides, sometimes termed neurotransmitters. This area of medicine, which is referred to as *psychoneuroimmunology*, suggests that chemicals produced in the brain and other sites have a profound effect on every part of the body via the receptors responding to these neurotramitters. Even thinking creates neuropeptides. Thus, this is truly mind over matter. The condition of illness or health certainly is in the patient's head, but it is activated at distant locations through these neuro-peptides and their receptors in various tissues. This dynamic represents a dialogue of sorts; the mind tells the tissues, and the tissues inform the mind.

What we think of as the meaning of our illness is also important. Past experiences and beliefs influence our historical neurochemistry, which either creates a balance, or in cases of "dis-ease," a dysfunction. An individual recognizes the constellation of symptoms in reference to his or her experience. It is not just the number of doctor visits or the specific treatments that make us better, but our relationship to, or our historical interpretation of, the illness. Thus, I frequently ask a patient what he feels is the significance of his medical problem.

Even when we try to listen to our bodies, they do not always speak clearly; they truly speak in metaphors, which require interpretation. People can, in fact, die of a broken heart, a mother can be a pain in the neck, and a job a pain in the ass! Certainly, these patients will complain of chest, neck, and sacroiliac pain. This may be a reflection of life's stresses and imposed disability. The symptoms of an illness therefore do have meaning, both literally and figuratively.

Given this interpretation of mind and matter, it's not what is scientifically proven, but what is intuitive for the patient that counts. So if the patient does not mind, it doesn't matter. Some illnesses, like trauma or heart attacks, are best treated by conventional orthodox medicines. Others, such as chronic pain syndrome, may best be treated by Chinese acupuncture or other unconventional medical philosophies. This is why I choose a holistic approach to treating a patient. I learned years ago that the average practitioner treats symptoms and a good doctor treats the disease, but the best physician treats the patient!

◆ ◆ ◆

"Treat people as though they were what they ought to be, and you will help them become what they are capable of being."

2

Twenty-First-Century Medicine

Dissatisfaction

Dissatisfaction encourages people to change. This was true even in the mythological origins of medicine. Asclepias, the son of Apollo, defied the gods and was struck down by Zeus for interfering with "divine" (often whimsical) order by relieving suffering and rescuing those stricken with death. His staff, on which the magical healing serpent ascends, is the emblem of our healing profession. Asclepias evokes the true heart of a physician, reminding us to have a personal bond with our patients and to make their individual welfare a prime consideration. For his compassion, skill, and dedication, Asclepias is mentioned in the Hippocratic Oath. This god should not, however, be confused with Hippocrates, the true father of modern medicine in whose honor medical school graduates take this oath. (See page 5.)

Like Asclepias, many physicians today are dissatisfied with the unquestioningly accepted limitations on healing taught in orthodox medical schools and postgraduate curricula. Counting myself among the disenchanted, I was privileged to hear James Gordon, MD, from Washington, DC, speak to a group of health professionals in Ann Arbor, Michigan. Much of the following is from this talk and his book, *The Manifesto of the New Medicine*.

Many conventional physicians have seen patients drift off increasingly to other "health care providers," both those

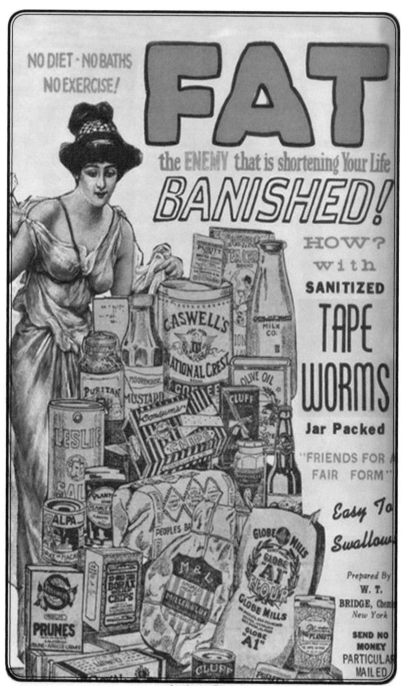

Antique Diet

who are qualified and those who are not. In a recent study, 54 percent of patients saw alternative practitioners in the twelve months preceding a visit to their medical doctor and, more importantly, less than half told their physicians about the other forms of treatment. Patients are clearly dissatisfied and, for that matter, so are physicians. A recent survey found that 36 percent of doctors said they would not go into medicine again if they were given the opportunity. Fortunately, the remaining 64 percent, like me, would do so again and again. Indeed, many of my colleagues are dropping out of medicine, not because the profession is too demanding, but because the standards of care and the medical bureaucracy have changed drastically. We no longer use thorough history-taking and physical examination for a clinical diagnosis. Instead, we make our diagnoses from expensive and frequently useless or dangerous tests, the byproducts of technological advancement.

Please do not misunderstand; I think technology enriches the health and welfare of all humankind. In our society, however, patients as well as doctors demand the latest tests, which frequently clarify nothing. Furthermore, the risks of many invasive testing procedures far outweigh the proposed benefits. The graduates of medical schools are not going into primary care, but the lucrative less frustrating specialties. That is why it is predicted that despite the prevalence of mid-level practitioners (physician assistants, PAs, advanced registered nurse practitioners, ARNPs), with the aging of the Baby Boomers there will be a true dearth of primary care physicians (PCPs).

A problem with orthodox medicine is that the focus of treatment is frequently obscured. Often the disease is treated, rather than the patient who suffers with the disorder. We were taught textbook cases of disease, but seldom do we see such a classic patient because there are many variations of a sickness. What happens in one individual with a certain illness may be completely different from another. Some patients have no symptoms while others have sub-clinical or non-specific ones, and, depending on the environment and constitutional background, still another could die from the same disease process. We as physicians may inherently know such a range of affliction exists, but it seldom enters into our therapeutic model of patient care. Most of us were taught that *"common diagnoses are common, and uncommon diagnoses are uncommon."* Yet, *uncommon* presentations of *common* diagnoses are far more *common* than *uncommon* diagnoses, but we do not apply this in our practices.

Until the first decade in the twentieth century, physicians incorporated the best of all known medical philosophies, combining homeopathic, herbal, ancient, and ultra-modern (e.g., electromagnetic) healing modalities in their practices. This was referred to as *eclectic medicine*. The problem with using such a variety of approaches was a lack of standards in both medical education and practice. Consequently, the Carnegie Foundation sponsored a commission, headed by the well-known academician Abraham Flexner. It published a report in 1910 that led to an almost instantaneous revision of the medical arts. Many of the commonly used methods were not scientifically supported and thus were cast out. Doctors using these therapeutic techniques were branded as quacks and charlatans. In the subsequent tidal wave of this mind-set, those healing therapies—many of which did have great value—have been slow to resurface. Now, even when scientific background accompanies their reemergence, these forms of healing are still not accepted by most mainstream physicians. In my opinion, however, the pendulum that was far to the left is swinging to the right.

The Cat Is Out of the Bag (CT Scan Kills)

CAT (Computer Axial Tomography) scans, now commonly called CT scans, are greatly over-ordered in the United States.

Given the highly profitable nature of diagnostic imaging, it's no wonder this procedure is overused. Costing roughly $600 per study for overhead (which includes office space, employees, and a radiologist) and the upkeep on the scanner (which includes the cost of and repairs to the unit when heavily used), but earning a $1500 reimbursement from the insurance companies, this procedure is lucrative. Some areas of the country do eight times more CT scans than other parts, yet they do not have any detectable increases in health—only more expense. (Americans pay more for health care than any other nation, yet we are thirty-second in health and longevity.) Moreover, when they are over-prescribed, CT scans are dangerous!

CT scans are risky in three ways. First, the patient is over-exposed to radiation. Second, it leads to more dangerous and unnecessary invasive procedures. Third, the contrast used with most of the scans damages the kidneys. In terms of radiation exposure, one CT scan equals up to 450 chest X-rays. This translates to an extra 30,000 cancers each year. Furthermore, radiation is cumulative and grows more each year. It may take twenty-five years for cancer to appear, but the mortality rate of these tumors, despite early detection and good treatment, is 50 percent.

The iodinated contrast material, which is injected into the veins for CT scans, is excreted by the kidneys. It is hypertonic and "dehydrates" the sensitive microvessels and tubules of this organ. Some of this tissue never fully recovers. Also 3 percent of the population is sensitive to these organic iodinated molecules. Very rarely can one encounter such an acute allergic reaction that causes death so suddenly! To avoid renal destruction, the radiologists should make sure the kidneys are working adequately by doing a serum BUN and creatinine, both of which are renal function tests. If the BUN is below 25, or the creatinine is less than 1.8, the contrast can be used for better definition. However even with normal function, unless the person is more than adequately hydrated and/or they take strong antioxidants such as N-acetyl cysteine, they will lose some kidney function every time they take the contrast. This is additive over the number of studies a patient has over their lifetime. N-Acetyl Cysteine (NAC), 600mg three times a day on the day before, the day of, and the day after the study, is advised. Lastly, CT scans are in many cases overly sensitive and can pick up incidental findings of no real clinical relevance. In other words, they may indicate a "false positive" of certain medical conditions. We use terms such as *incidentaloma* for so-called tumors that have no clinical manifestions and should be left alone, but are yet aggressively treated like a malevolent malignancy. Our medical profession should "let sleeping dogs lie" in many of these cases, but they do not for reasons that may not be purely altruistic.

The medical mind-set taught to young doctors is *the more, the better* in our land of plenty. In actuality, this approach makes more money for physicians by increasing the number of procedures and operations they participate in or encourage. On the other hand, this leads to heightened anxiety and unnecessary testing, biopsies, and even surgeries, creating earlier disability and death for the patient. With new health care legislation around the corner, the problem will only get worse. Because most patients are not told the full extent of the risks and consequences of these procedures, they are ultimately frightened into invasive actions that are unnecessary.

The Law of Consequences

As I mentioned earlier, it is not *who* is right but *what* is right that counts. This statement is based in part on a natural law that operates in the universe called "The Law of Consequences": Every action will have a reaction, and for every act we perform there is a natural and appropriate consequence. What follows in this section comes not from research, but from my heart.

I feel sorry for many people I see in the news each day. The radio, television, Internet, and newspapers are filled with stories of those who either didn't know about the "Law of Consequences," or thought it would not catch up with them when they committed immoral, unethical, or illegal acts.

Unfortunately, these folks failed to realize they were sowing seeds that would sooner or later come up, exposing selfishness and corruption for all to see. Even if their malicious actions were never revealed, dark secrets take an even greater toll. For instance, we can never escape from who we really are or the consequences of our actions. When we commit a serious misdeed, its malignancy stays with us as long as we live, and afterward in our soul and even to our progeny.

On the other hand, while all pernicious acts consume life, all just and compassionate ones nurture and renew it. In this sense, the law of consequences allows us to tell our own fortunes. When our actions are based on truth, honesty, and integrity, over time good things will come to us. This is not to say that bad things do not happen to good people. We all know they do. When we face hardship or injury we need not ask, "Why me?" but rather, "How will I respond?" If one has a good heart there are no mistakes, only lessons. We will learn and grow from our misfortune.

The earth can provide for our need, but not for our greed. Egocentrism teases us with immediate and tangible results, but altruism is more fulfilling and rewarding. Many good people fail to realize all the blessings they can receive from being of service to others. If we look for ways to help other people, with the right attitude and the right motive, more good will come our way than we ever dreamed possible. Broadcast optimistic thoughts, talk, and actions. The Law of Sowing and Reaping is clear: "Don't sow wild oats and pray for crop failure." You will get what you give.

Table 2-I

Alternative Therapies

Acupuncture
Applied Kinesiology
Aromatherapy
Ayurvedic Medicine
Biofeedback Training
Biological Dentistry
Bodywork
Botanical Medicine
Chelation Therapy
Chiropractic
Colon Therapy
Craniosacral Therapy
Detoxification Therapy
Diet Therapy
Electrical Therapy
Energy Medicine
Environmental Medicine
Enzyme Medicine
Fasting
Flower Remedies
Guided Imagery
Homeopathy
Iridology
Juice Therapy

Kinergetics
Light Therapy
Live Cell Therapy (Thymus)
Magnetic Field Therapy
Massage Therapy
Meditation
Mind/Body Medicine
Motion Therapy
Naturopathic Medicine
Neural Therapy
Neuro-Linguistic Programming
Nutritional Supplements
Orthomolecular Medicine
Osteopathy
Oxygen Therapy
Ozone Therapy
Qigong
Reconstructive Therapy
Reicke
Reflexology
Sound Therapy
Touch Therapy
Traditional Chinese Medicine
Yoga

The above is a partial list. Other healing treatments have been described, and there are several sub-categories of most of those listed.

An Antidote to Antibiotics

Health care consumers are voting with their wallets, choosing to spend more health care dollars on supplements and alternative medicine than on traditional care, even though it may be subsidized by third-party carriers. This trend is admirable and hopefully will decrease some of the problems we are having with microbial resistance to the antibiotics on the market now, as well as those in the future. Practicing community physicians stand accused of abusing rather than using antibiotics appropriately. Hence they are blamed for the increasing microbial resistance that the modern world is experiencing. This incidental overprescribing, however, represents only the tip of the iceberg.

A significant factor associated with bacterial resistance is increased antibiotic use in hospitals where these drugs are used empirically, rather than after bacterial cultures and sensitivities to the drug are obtained. Instead of using a narrow spectrum antibiotic for a specific bug, many hospitalists use a broad spectrum drug. Repeated antibiotic courses and prolonged hospitalizations compound the problem. The hospital ecology and the immuno-compromised patient cause antibiotic resistance. Increased use of invasive devices and catheters, ineffective infection control procedures, and intra-hospital transfers of colonized patients are other factors.

International travel has been implicated in the problem, but the real culprit is animal husbandry and agricultural use. Annually in the United States, approximately ten million kg of anti-microbial agents are used for animals and twenty-five thousand kg are used for fruit trees. The antibiotics used in agrifood industries are numerous, including chlortetracycline, erythromycin, bactracin, penicillin, streptomycin, and lincomycin. Antibiotics engineered for animals and plants usually precede those used for humans and fight many of the same bacteria that infect humans. This allows the development of bacteria already resistant when the drug is finally approved for human use. Many veterinarian drugs, such as sarafloxacin, are very closely related to those used in humans, like ciprofloxacin. Vancomycin resistance in our hospitals of staph and enterococci is already here. If enough consumers will demand organic foods, this problem can be reduced. If one does use an antibiotic, concomitant probiotics (friendly intestinal bacteria) should be ingested. This is done with the first antibiotic dose and carried on for three days afterward.

Using herbal and complementary medicine techniques to boost a person's immune defense will decrease antibiotic usage, thereby limiting the emergence of resistant bacteria strains. The development of antiviral agents, which is coming at an incredible pace, will supplement this process. So I advise not taking an antibiotic for a minor infection that is, more likely than not, viral. Children, perhaps at the parents' insistence, are often given antibiotics for trivial reasons. While this is good for the pharmaceutical companies, it is bad for both the patient and our planet.

Combined Medicine

We should treat folks by boosting the immune system with inexpensive plant-based supplements. Spirulena, echinacea, golden seal, and sacchomyces cervacea are just a few safe, inexpensive, and effective supplements that are available. As mentioned before, we are starting to swing from mainstream medicine to *alternative medicine*. *Alternative* means "other than." This includes everything that we medical students did not learn in school and what is not customarily practiced in our clinics and hospitals. In the last several years, some of us may have been discovering what we did not learn in our formal studies. The good news is that recently some medical schools have added alternative therapies (see Figure II-2) to their curriculums. *Complementary medicine,* a British term, indicates those alternatives that can complement, or add to, conventional medicine.

Holistic medicine is a term that was first used in Western scientific literature in 1926 by Jan Christian Smuts, a South African biologist and statesman who wrote the book *Holism and Evolution.* The term comes from the Greek word *holos,* for "whole." The concept is that the whole is greater than the sum of its parts. This is as true of organisms as it is of communities.

On the other hand, Bacon and Descartes, famous philosophers of the sixteenth century, believed that to know an organism one must dissect and understand it in progressively smaller parts. Through this kind of analysis, they declared, we can know the whole truth of a living creature. Kurt Goldstine, MD, offered yet another thesis that was perhaps more germane: the *organistic theory.* He was a well-known psychiatrist who worked with men who had been brain-damaged in World War I due to trauma. Dr. Goldstine found that, contrary to some of the outstanding research done previously in brain localization and function of the body, most patients who had major portions of their brains shot away—parts that were supposedly responsible for particular actions—were still able to carry out those functions, demonstrating the brain's capacity to reorganize itself and the premise of holistic medicine. (Kirlean photography demonstrates this: Cut a leaf in half, photograph it with this technique, and the other half appears.) This idea began in 1922, but only a few biologists espoused it until the 1970s. In 2008, a well-studied patient who had two centimeters of brain surgically removed in 1964 for seizures, was autopsied, and it confirmed this theory. His seizures ceased after his surgery, but so did his memory. He could not remember anything that was from more than five minutes previous. The whole *is* greater than its parts.

The lay definition of holistic medicine today includes the entire field of various non-orthodox medical healing

If a Dog Were Your Teacher, You would learn...

When loved ones come home, always run to greet them.

Never pass up the opportunity to go for a joyride.

Allow the experience of fresh air and the wind in your face to be pure ecstasy.

When it's in your best interest — practice obedience.

Let others know when they've invaded your territory.

Take naps and stretch before rising.

Run, romp and play daily.

Thrive on attention and let people touch you.

Avoid biting, when a simple growl will do.

On warm days, stop to lie on your back on the grass.

On hot days, drink lots of water and lie under a shady tree.

No matter how often you're scolded, don't buy into the guilt thing and pout ... run right back and make friends.

Delight in the simple joy of a long walk.

Eat with gusto and enthusiasm.

Stop when you have had enough.

Be loyal.

Never pretend to be something you're not.

If what you want lies buried, dig until you find it.

When someone is having a bad day, be silent, sit close by and nuzzle them gently.

procedures such as acupuncture or magnetic therapy, as well as orthodox academic medicine. The holistic physician will use whatever it takes—conventional, eclectic, and prayer—to heal the patient. If a few pills a day of the inexpensive and safe Saw Palmetto will shrink an enlarged prostate, why give a more expensive drug with possible side effects such as Avodart? On the other hand, if one has bacterial pneumonia, a real antibiotic is needed, not Colloidal Silver or Echinacea. However, a true holistic doctor may use both the herb and the drug to augment their healing potential.

Mind-body medicine was briefly discussed earlier. It emphasizes the effects of the mind on the body and vice versa. The complete interaction of mind over body is well known, but the reverse is not. The discovery in the 1940s of neurotransmitters established that the body could indeed talk to the mind as much as the brain could communicate with the body. An all-inclusive moniker might be, in the German style of word grafting, *psychoneuroimmunoendocrinology.* Although that might be a mouthful, research has revealed that the very same receptors and neurotransmitters are present in and around the cells of the brain, the endocrine system, peripheral nervous and immune systems, the intestinal system, and all organs of the body. Such an approach provides for ongoing feedback among virtually each part of every organ of the body. Mind-body medicine seeks to enter this conversation and improve the level of discourse of the entire human being.

There is more grey matter, the neurons that make neurotransmitters, below the neck than above. It is said that the intestine has a mind of its own and is sometimes contrary. I have a patient who has no desire to have a bowel movement while at home, but as soon as she leaves the house, it comes on mightily! The mind does enhance both physical and psychological well-being. The same neurotransmitters do work in reverse, and detract modulating, for better or worse, mood and mental functioning.

Integrative Medicine technically has a different connotation than holistic medicine. It involves integrating different healing modalities and healing systems into mainstream medicine, including the essences of primitive, ancient, arcane, and other healing paradigms. Examples of primitive forms of healing are acupuncture and herbology, which date back to the caveman. Ayurvedic (continental Indian) and Chinese traditional medicine illustrate ancient forms of the healing arts that, indeed, worked. Homeopathy is considered an arcane form, along with natural and electromagnetic vibrational energy transference and barometric/weather medicine. Integrative medicine also draws on chiropractic and various forms of mind-body healing, such as meditation, hypnosis, and religion. Healing by faith has existed for five millennia and, in my opinion, will continue until the end of time. Accordingly, integrative medicine can also bridge the gap between conventional Western medicine and non-conventional healing. It puts the patient in the driver's seat *and* partners with them.

New medicine is a useful term and may be synonymous with the best of medicine. For the first time on this planet we have the opportunity and the inclination to integrate these many approaches. The breed that emerges from this manifold fertilization is the *New Medicine*. We now understand the healing arts that have been used in various cultures throughout time and incorporate them into our practices. Though these other disciplines are not new, bringing them together with Western science is. I also like the term *New Medicine* because it never goes out of date; what is new is always evolving, and medicine should, too.

Consider the transformation of what we now think of as modern medicine. More and more research for chronic illness concludes there are no "magic bullets," a term coined by the great physician, Paul Ehrlich, who found, in the 1890s, a "cure" for syphilis. When physicians were using an arsenic compound for the disease, arsenic was thought to be a godsend. But as the months and years rolled on, some patients became fatally ill because of the treatment; the cure was worse than the disease. The concept has evolved, and some "bullets," although not magic, do indeed help—like using antibiotics for bacterial infections. Still, some of these "bullets" start ricocheting, producing antibiotic resistant bacteria such as MRSA Occasionally, we are no better at treating certain infections than we were in Dr. Ehrlich's time. However, using the best of the old, the recent, and the forthcoming, the *New Medicine* can help our patients far more than the so-called standard or allopathic medicine alone.

The lack of individuality, partnership, and self-care in today's medical system also drives us toward the *New Medicine*. One has to look no further than the celebrated Patch Adams for the individual practice philosophy in physician-patient relationships. It is well-documented that being lighthearted and happy uniquely improves our immune systems. Perhaps Norman Cousins was correct when he wrote his book, *Laughter Is the Best Medicine*. There are, understandably, peculiarities that bring those giving care and those seeking it together. Most patients who come to my practice do so because they want an approach that they feel will be more successful than what they have received. Frequently, they want a method that will help them feel better while another therapy takes hold, such as giving a potent anti-inflammatory for acute rheumatoid arthritis while waiting for a disease-modifying agent to take effect. Another example is cancer patients undergoing radiation and chemotherapy that may get rid of the cancer, but what about their health and well-being while the treatments are ongoing? Patients are miserable, fatigued, and without immunity. Inevitably, patients come to the *New Medicine* for alternatives, and find the doctors actually spending time listening to them. This *New Medicine* is what is visualized on TV, not just the old *Marcus Welby* approach, but also on the recent show *House*.

A major factor in switching health care philosophies is that patients believe they will receive more care from doctors who say they are holistic, alternative, complementary, or integrated because these practitioners will take more time and pay more attention to other aspects of a patient's life. For example, the use of supplements with radiation and conventional oncology or in cases of extremely resistant cancers, supplements altogether and no further medical treatment, may be best for the patient. It is hard for an oncologist to accept that. I once asked a colleague when he usually stops chemotherapy. His reply was "When the patient gets too sick from his chemotherapy, dies, or when his insurance runs out."

Another major force driving this mild revolution is health maintenance organizations (HMOs). They are maintaining but not enhancing people's health by preventing disease. Furthermore, the less time health professionals have for people under the guise of efficiency, the more the patients resent that system. Some HMOs and insurance companies are starting to allow for alternative medicine. This results in more satisfaction for the patient, less expense for diagnosis and treatment, and future savings by delaying or preventing a disease. Their real concern is continued return: An HMO or insurance company may carry a patient this year, but not the next. Thus, the organization is reluctant to pay for the prevention of a disease process for a patient who may switch to another company at any time. These institutions are finding out that in addition to giving the patient more satisfaction now, the *New Medicine* physician does, in fact, practice more prevention than conventional doctors do. This will save the company more money in the long run, no matter who benefits today.

In the last few years Medicare has started paying for a one-time "Welcome to Medicare" exam with lipids, chemistries, EKGs, paps, mammographies, etc., and an annual health care screen. In the near future it will pay primary care doctors (PCPs) more for each patient if they have an office that will manage the patients' "preventive" care, such as flu vaccinations, pap tests, and even colonoscopy procedures when needed.

As a result of our information revolution, patients and their families are becoming more knowledgeable. They have access to medical information through TV, the Internet, popular magazines, books, newsletters, and word of mouth. (Many physicians have their own websites. Mine is www.docblock.com.) EMR (Electronic Medical Records) will be mandatory for physicians starting in 2012. E-Scripts, transmission of records, and laboratory follow-up will be performed with a click of the mouse. Aptly, this medical crisis holds both the danger of a reactionary limiting of health care, as well as a revolutionary opportunity to save money and lives by working with an amalgamated system of the *New Medicine*. Although this is very different from the orthodox medical program most of us were taught, I feel the *New Medicine* is here to stay and, in time, it may outdistance the arrows of the doubting allopathic physician.

Some established and well-seasoned aspects of healing have proven to be effective not only for decades or centuries, but millennia. The *New Medicine* physician selects the best from all these disciplines using, for example: acupuncture from Chinese medicine, electromagnetic diagnosis from energy medicine, remedies from homeopathic medicine, and echinacea from herbal medicine, all for a particular patient—with no system being exclusive. Some of these approaches may have been mentioned briefly in medical school, but usually in a derogatory sense. It is about time that we start teaching these precepts in the curricula of all medical schools as we now teach nutrition. But that is only part of the solution.

Practicing physicians are resistant, and practice habits are hard to change. Unfortunately, the enlightened physician is frequently ridiculed to the point that he is considered to be using a lower standard of care by his colleagues. They may even report him to the state licensing board, especially if he is very successful in his practice. In the coming years the medical community, especially the most entrenched and pharisaical physicians, will have to accept this metamorphosis. Then I, and others like me, including patients and other health professionals, shall live in peace and harmony with one another as medical colleagues.

Intuitively we understand that we are all unique. We also know we have many minute differences such as blood type, IQ, and influences by certain foods. In the first year or two of medical school, we are taught to spend enough time in our initial encounter with a patient to get to know him or her intimately. Some still do, initially, but most never spend that much time with a patient again! With more continued one-on-one time, it becomes easier to know the uniqueness of that person and to focus on how that person fits into certain diagnostic categories by considering the emotional, environmental, physical, and laboratory findings. In many primary care practices, lab tests are done before the patient even sees a doctor. It is not just a convenience that the initial focus is on a lab test rather than on the individual; it is a sign of the times. Why not figure out first which lab tests, if any, are really needed? Then, if a lab test does not agree with a patient's diagnosis, throw out the lab test, not the patient. The test should confirm or refute the working diagnosis and not give information that could be, and often is, wrong. We need to treat the patient, not the lab test. The point is that each person is not only psychologically but also biologically unique! Dr. Roger Williams, the innovator of a cellular micronutient test noted below, discovered this principle.

Micronutrient (vitamins, amino acids, minerals, anti-oxidants, metabolites) deficiencies contribute to the broad range of minor and serious health conditions. Identifying and correcting them is an important component of management and/or treatment of cardiovascular disease, diabetes, cancer, osteoporosis, chronic fatigue, and other so-called chronic degenerative conditions like osteoarthritis. *The Journal of the American Medical Association* in an article titled "Vitamins for Chronic Disease Prevention in Adults," states: "Although clinical syndromes of vitamin deficiencies are unusual in Western societies, suboptimal status is not." There are many serum nutritional tests but they only measure static quantities of vitamins and minerals present in serum, such as magnesium or B12 reflecting dietary intake and not what *cannot* get into our cells rather than the true cellular content and function. But there is a test that can assess long-term intracellular requirements using each patient's own lymphocytes. Under a variety of nutrient depletion conditions, scientists can now measure the growth response of these cells to something called mitogenic stimulation. This determines intracellular deficiencies, which might not be detected by standard serum tests, giving us a true window on intracellular function.

In 1949, Dr. Roger Williams, who previously discovered five vitamins, coined the word *genetotrophic* disease, which means having both genetic (*geneto*) and nutritional (*trophic*) roots. Later (1956) he published the book *Biochemical Individuality: The Basis for the Genetotrophic Concept*. William Shive, PhD, who was chairman of the department of biochemistry and a researcher in the field of nutrition at the University of Texas, began work on a diagnostic test for clinicians in 1978. His work was strongly influenced by Roger Williams, PhD. Dr. Shive first identified appropriate cells for the functional assays. He selected lymphocyte cells because they are simple to collect (via venipuncture), easily isolated from other whole blood components, and maintainable in culture for days to weeks.

These harvested lymphocytes are in a resting state in terms of cell division. Since they have a four to six-month lifespan, the nutrient levels accumulated in these lymphocytes represent a history of an individual's nutrient status. This is analogous to using HbA1c measurements to approximate a diabetic person's glucose levels over the preceding three months. Thus, lymphocytes provide a history rather than a snapshot of nutrient intake. Resting lymphocytes can be stimulated by a lymphocyte-specific mitogen to undergo cell division and grow in culture. The degree of growth that the lymphocytes can maintain is directly related to the nutrients they have available. The cells are stimulated to grow in the control media containing optimal amounts of specific micronutrients. As each micronutrient is removed from the media, the cells must use their own internal mechanisms (reserves or metabolic processes) to grow. If cells grow optimally, they are functioning adequately and thus are not deficient. If cells do not grow optimally, then a deficiency is indicated. For example, when zinc is removed from the media and cell growth is not sufficient, this indicates that the lymphocyte cells have a *functional intracellular* deficiency of zinc.

A functional deficiency encompasses any of the factors that reduce the efficacy of a nutrient. Thus, a given nutrient may be present, but it may not be properly activated, be appropriately localized, or have sufficient cofactors to function at a normal level of activity. Whatever the cause, the result will be a defect in the biochemical pathways that depend upon that nutrient for optimal function. A deficient or defective pathway may operate at a sub-optimal level for many months, or even years, before a clinical symptom becomes apparent.

Micronutrient deficiencies aren't just a reflection of diet. Since we are all biochemically unique, nutrient deficiencies will vary from person to person, and do not necessarily correlate directly with nutrient intake, even among those with similar health conditions. Many factors beyond diet determine whether nutrient function is adequate. These include biochemical individuality, genetic predisposition, absorption and metabolism, age, disease conditions, and medications. Some folks spend hundreds of dollars a year and don't need to. Others need a few inexpensive supplements to stay healthy, and this test details the best for each of us. This is personal medicine at its highest level, rather than what most of us doctors practice: "One Size Fits All."

One can be deficient in micronutrients and not even know it until it is too late and, for example, develop cancer. Studies have shown that 50 percent of patients taking a multivitamin are functionally deficient in one or more essential nutrients that are vital to long-term health. Deficiencies suppress the function of the immune system and contribute to degenerative processes. *Propetology* is another word coined by Dr. Williams, which is the potential science of the "leaning" (Greek) of individuals toward certain diseases. This is a genetic or other predisposing factor that gives one person the tendency to have a given medical problem, but another with the same exposure may not have any difficulty.

Spectrox is a total antioxidant function test that assesses the ability of cells to resist damage caused by free radicals and other forms of oxidative stress that is included in the study using the same technology as the micronutrient testing.

The micronutrient test was prohibitively expensive until recently, when it began to be produced commercially by Spectracell Laboratories. (Spectracell is the descendant company of Drs. Williams and Shive.) This test is paid for by most insurance companies, including Medicare and Medicaid, except for a $160 copay.

Comprehensive Nutritional Panel

Vitamins	Minerals	Amino Acids	Antioxidants	Carbohydrate Metabolism, Fatty Acids & Metabolites
Biotin	Calcium	Asparagine	Lipoic Acid	Carnitine
Folate	Copper	Glutamine	Coenzyme Q10	Choline
Pantothenate	Magnesium	Serine	Cysteine	Chromium
Vitamin A	Zinc		Glutathione	Fructose Sensitivity
Vitamin B1			Selenium	Glucose/Insulin Metabolism
Vitamin B2			Vitamin E	Inositol
Vitamin B3			SPECTROX™ (Total Antioxidant Function)	Oleic Acid
Vitamin B6				
Vitamin B12				
Vitamin C				
Vitamin D				
Vitamin K2				

Normal Is Not Optimal

Lab values of personal health requirements are only rough estimates of a statistical average. Thus, they do not invariably apply to a given individual who presents with a particular symptom complex. For example, we use averages, such as the RDAs for nutrition. As noted above, Dr. Roger Williams spent the last forty-five years of his life studying our biochemical individuality and learning that we differ by as much as thirty-fold in our need for certain nutrients. Even with the same basic weight, age, and medical history, one may need thirty times as much zinc as another, or thirty times as much B6 or folic acid to produce a certain enzymatic reaction, based on the genetic and environmental variance of need for any given person.

Normal laboratory values are derived from testing a large number of *presumably* healthy individuals and plotting their laboratory results in a bell-shaped curve. Values within two standard deviations of the mean are accepted as "normal." This is a statistical term that should, by definition, apply to 87.5 percent of the population. By my definition, a value is no longer optimal when it reaches any level where risk starts to adversely affect function. This is quite different from just being in the statistical range that most doctors consider normal.

The definition of *normal* is also influenced by technology. Laboratory examinations have been available to patients since the ancient days of medicine. Not very sophisticated in their earliest forms, they consisted of diagnosing diabetes by tasting a patient's urine to determine the presence of sugar. Today laboratory tests range from basic bacterial cultures and routine chemistry panels to highly complex immunologically derived processes. All are intended to determine the presence or absence of an underlying disease state. For example, in the early days of measuring cholesterol, we accepted total values as high as 330 mg/dl as normal, and now it is less than 200. Once we achieved the ability to measure fractions of cholesterol, we began thinking of the *lousy* LDL of less than 130 MG/dl and *healthy* HDL greater than 45 as normal. With **ADVANCE LIPID TESTING** we can now split out the neutral LDL from the small dense LDL along with the Remanant Particles that *really* narrows our arteries. Likewise, the active HDL 2 from the inert HDL 3 that better determines the health of our blood vessels.

Some physicians have already adjusted their interpretation and lab results to reflect optimal values. Now, an LDL level of less than 100 is considered most efficacious for cardiovascular health. A complete cardiovascular risk panel—including Homocysteine, HsCRP, Fibrogen, Apolipoprotein E, Uric Acid, A1C-Hg, MPO, Plac-2, Fast Calcium CT scan, Thalum tread-mill, and clotting factors—predicts far better the patient's cardiovascular health. Even with this more detailed analysis, referring only to a range of normal results may create an illusion that the individual is fine. Many experienced physicians know that a patient on the fringes of the range is not as healthy as one in the middle. For example, a person with a potassium level of 3.5—within the normal range of 3.5 to 5—is much more likely to have a fatal heart arrhythmia than if the value was 4.2. A fifty-year-old male feels and performs better with a testosterone level of 800 than 300, even though both are in the normal range of 300 to 1,000. Although the normal range of the thyroid test TSH is 0.5 to 5.5, the patient does far better if it is between 0.5 and 1.7. Thus, lab results should be interpreted for optimal values that inform the individual of the possible need of dietary supplements, antioxidants, hormones, or pharmaceuticals. This approach gives the knowledgeable physician more effective tools for establishing goals and managing the patient's individual health program. Do not hesitate to discuss optimal versus normal values with your doctor.

The Placebo Effect

Doctors should try to make the best therapeutic decisions for their patients by using evidence-based medicine along with their medical judgment. However, the physician's real success depends on their attitude, demeanor, personality, time spent with the patient, ability to communicate, and most importantly, commitment to help. These are the elements of a good doctor/patient relationship, which is being eroded these days by pressures from third-party payers, lawyers, politicians, and fragmented care from specialists.

Medicine is actually an art based on science. The placebo works well in chronic, painful, benign disorders that have no actual pathology, or that will heal themselves with time. It also works better on those who have high expectations of the medication or procedure and, most of all, the physician's demeanor. Surprisingly, a favorable attitude toward the physician by the patient was not part of the placebo responder. Contrary to popular belief, educated people, professionals, working women, nonsmokers, and farmers were more likely to respond to the placebo. These folks are usually self-sufficient individuals and unaccustomed to dependency. A person may respond to a placebo sometimes and not others. Sufficient time for the doctor to talk to the patient personally, as well as the disease process, is directly correlated to the patient's success with a placebo. This may be why a formal homeopath who knows well the patient after two hours of interview does so well with inert "drugs."

Colds get better on their own, but terminal cancer does not, and it is the least susceptible to the placebo effect. However, I have witnessed actual "cures" in cancer patients by treatments other doctors would consider "placebos," such as vibrational therapy (Rife Light), and herbs. Placebos answer the human need for care when feeling ill, and this certainly can be achieved without prejudice or deception. In primary care, half the patients have complaints that don't lend themselves to a definite diagnosis. For these, specific medications do not work. It is a trial-and-error process until the doctor finds something that will help. But even if a physician cannot cure a patient, they can at least care. Compassion, encouragement, a positive attitude, and involved time with the patient go a long way, even if the doctor knows there may be no effective medical treatment. Our fragmented modern health care system fosters the "nocebo" (not to please), rather than the "placebo" (to please). The disease in the patient is treated rather than the patient with the disease. Surely we physicians can do better.

Evidence-Based Medicine

EBM is a new paradigm that has brought a better clarity of diagnosis and treatment to the medical community. Previously, physicians would use anecdotal information, personal experience, inductive reasoning concerning pathophysiology of disease, previous teaching, and tremendous prejudice and biases for clinical decisions. What was thought of, but not really documented as true, is still practiced by most doctors.

This includes old wives' tales and consensus opinion. The latter was obtained when a committee of experts in a field voted on how to diagnosis and treat. There is a gap of years, if not decades, between clinical research and clinical practice. We need to enhance clinical decision trees, utilizing theory and better statistical modeling.

Levels of Evidence for EBM

The *New Medicine* emphasizes the patient's preferences based on their value system and beliefs. Moreover we encourage patients to do their own quality searches of EBM. Doctors are discouraged from using their beliefs and value systems, but encouraged to be "objective." Archie Cochrane's 1972 book, *Effectiveness and Efficiency: Random Reflections on Health Services,* advocated computerized literature. This is now a reality. Scientific studies are included in the *Cochrane Database* which,

Ia	Meta-analysis of randomized controlled trials
Ib	At least one randomized controlled trial
IIa	At least one well-designed, controlled study, but without randomization
IIb	At least one well-designed quasi-experimental study
III	At least one-non-experimental descriptive study (eg. comparative, correlation or case-controlled study)
IV	Expert committee reports, opinions and/or experiences of respected authorities
V	Anecdotal accounts of multiple patient outcomes from a particular therapy

as of 2010, has over 3,500 systemic reviews and is still growing. It is easily accessible to both doctors and their patients. Medline.com and PubMed.com are just several medical information sites obtained by browsing on the Internet.

EBM is a process in evaluation. Guidelines for treatment are being worked into the fabric of everyday clinical practice. With the advent of electronic medical records, EBM is being used to assess the quality of care by third-party payers, which give demerits to those not adhering to their recommendations and financial bonuses for those who do. There is a growing discontent among gifted clinicians who realize that some of these studies are funded by Big Pharma and are significantly skewed in favor of pharmaceutical organizations, thereby protecting profits. The government has its own agenda. Politicians speak of efficiency and cost-saving from the biases of the "scientists" who were trained at an institution and imbued with the government and the drug companies' philosophies.

Out-of-the-Box Thinking

There are a few of us who still think out of the box. These innovative physicians are well aware of the literature but, because of dumb luck or divine intervention, they derive a novel set of physical findings or laboratory tests. They give a different spin to a disease with a better diagnostic acumen or treatment of a malady. New diseases or new treatments for old diseases are discovered all the time, but in conventional medicine, where "one size fits all," they are largely ignored. There is as much variability metabolically and in the presentation of the disease as there is inconsistency in facial appearances. It is the *patient with the disease*, rather than the *disease in the patient*, who needs to be diagnosed and treated that makes all the difference in good patient care. It takes a strong backbone, however, for a doctor to stand up against organized medicine and maintain his/her dignity. Do not choose a physician who is too far out of the box and ignores, or is ignorant of, conventional wisdom. Pick one who knows what other doctors know, but who is willing to go one step beyond.

Discontentment and Disease

Many of us are tremendously dissatisfied, not only with our society, but in particular, with our work. Part of our process of healing, whether it is from heart disease, infection, or even cancer, has to do with profoundly changing some or all aspects of our lives. For example, our workplaces, the way we work, or even the particular kind of work we do could be detrimental. As with my colleagues in their primary care medical practices, about 60 percent of my patients have serious problems with their occupations. One must deal with these issues. They are major factors in overall health. Consider an unhappy paralegal who is word-processing all day long. While she works, she is cursing the boss for how much work she has to do. She is, indeed, in a stressful situation.

Much of her neuroendobiology is in overdrive, causing an internal imbalance. She will likely develop some malady such as carpal tunnel syndrome, a stiff neck, or pain in her shoulders or lower back because she is rigid and furious. I have some patients who are writers, and none of them ever have carpal tunnel syndrome. These folks spend as much time at the word processor as the paralegal, but they like their work. Of course, not every administrative assistant develops the syndrome, but the ones I have met who do, tend to be very dissatisfied with their work. So, how can I help her? Therapy may include vitamin B6, acupuncture, hypnosis, a local steroid injection, or even surgery for her carpal tunnel syndrome. These do not, however, address the underlying problem of her dissatisfaction; they just apply a Band-Aid to the issue. A good practitioner needs to consider all aspects of the patient in the whole of the healing scheme. According to a published study of men in Massachusetts, the major cause of first heart attacks was not heredity, high cholesterol, hypertension, or smoking, but rather job dissatisfaction.

George Angle, a professor of medicine at the University of Rochester, wrote several books in the 1960s on the fundamental causes of illness. Over a period of many years, he considered patients with a variety of serious illnesses, including cancer, heart disease, stroke, multiple sclerosis, and Parkinson's disease. When he went back and took histories of these people, he found that in the years before the onset of illness many described a sense of giving up. Eighty percent of the people who developed these serious, often life-threatening illnesses felt they were losing, or had already lost, the game of life. These patients were adults, many of them professionals, not children who could be easily influenced. When Angle went back to their families to make sure this was not some kind of retrospective bias, he confirmed his hypothesis: Disease is caused by *dis-ease!*

Unhappy people are prone to major illness. This conclusion is closely related to the mind-body interaction discussed earlier. We know, for example, the mind affects our immune system. A depressed immune system is fertile ground not only for infection, but also cancer. If the immune system is overstimulated, inflammatory diseases such as rheumatoid arthritis or coronary artery disease can occur. So, in addition to conventional histories, physicals, and lab studies, a patient's condition of ease or perspective on his or her own life needs to be considered. This is the holistic approach found in the *New Medicine.*

Traditionally, the spiritual dimension or the need for a spiritual advisor is mentioned only when a patient is close to death. At that point the chaplain is called in. Otherwise, the spiritual aspect is more or less ignored and even factored out of total health care. In a good medical practice, however, we do not have to abide by this taboo. I have seen faith's effect on both health and illness. I also pray with and for my patients. Mercifully we have seen miracles. Patients thank me, but I thank Him!

The Internal Healer

This new medicine should emphasize the healing within. This practice is commonly used by psychotherapists, but not by primary care physicians. The patient and the doctor need a therapeutic alliance. The benefit of an alliance is fortification, in this context, against disease. Dr. Bernie Siegel, the famous cancer surgeon, has his patients use a combat metaphor with imaging. He asks them to see in their mind's eye the artillery of chemotherapy raining down and destroying the cancer. If they have an infection, he has them visualize the white cells amassing and invading the bacteria. In his books he gives numerous examples of how we can best practice the art of imagery. Rather than being passive, we can learn about an illness and its vulnerable areas and attack the disease. This mobilizes the whole human system and favorably affects the outcome. This healing partnership implies collaboration, not compliance. You are working with your doctor, not just following his orders.

In many doctor-patient relationships, *compliance* is an ugly word. It means, "You do what I tell you; and if you do, you are a good patient, and if you do not, you are a bad patient!" I prefer to be in league with my patients. We're on the same team. As I mentioned earlier, I am the coach, he or she is the captain, and, together, the team makes the essential decisions about treatment. The patient may obtain most of the information from me, but I also urge him or her to consult other individuals, a support group, the Internet, books, and magazine articles about the illness. I encourage my patients to discuss those things with me, and I frequently learn from them. This kind of personal research is important to the partnership because a person who is completely involved with the disease, and who more or less understands the treatment, will do what is recommended with conviction, rather than simply out of compliance with what the doctor thinks is right. Two doctors, three opinions, but the opinion that really counts is the patient's. It is the patient, not the physician, who will pay the price for making the wrong diagnosis or being treated for the right disease but with an inappropriate therapy. Over-treatment may be worse than under-treatment. As a doctor I will do my best to help overcome the malady, but the patient has the responsibility for his disease; he owns it and he is the one who must live with it. At times, a patient requests a particular therapy even when I think another is better. Many times I act as a facilitator, helping them in the way they handle the disease. Many times the patient's choice is better than mine would have been.

Unfortunately, this type of patient involvement or self-care is neglected in today's medical philosophy. Self-care includes learning about ourselves, as well as taking care of ourselves. Then we can expand our knowledge and help others to take care of themselves. Self-care must encompass self-awareness; we must have a sense of what is going on before we can do something about it. I ask people, "Why do you think this is happening? Why do you think you had five colds this winter when you never had more than one before this? Why is your blood pressure suddenly skyrocketing at this time?" After patients get over their initial shock—"This is what I came here to find out"— most of them can tell me that something has changed: things are terrible at home; they hate their work supervisor; they are depressed; they are eating too much because they are stressed; and so on. Whatever it might be, they usually do have a sense of what went wrong and, hence, precipitated their medical problem. This is discovering the physician within.

RELAXATION

Learning how to relax is basic to self-care. Relaxation is the antidote for stress, the fight-or-flight response. It is a balancing of an involuntary wrestling match between the parasympathetic and the sympathetic nervous systems. True relaxation is a form of concentrated meditation that changes our brain waves from the *beta*, or active thinking state, to the *alpha*, which is the relaxed state. If we can get ourselves into a relaxed state for ten to twenty minutes twice a day, we can change virtually every physiological function in our bodies, and, as a result, improve our physical and mental condition. When we temporarily eliminate the mental tug-of-war in our daily routines and allow the body to enter a state of quiet counterpoise, our natural homeostasis, balance, and functional equilibrium begins to prevail. Many techniques are used to foster relaxation; several simple ones follow.

Sit comfortably in a quiet room in a chair and uncross your legs and arms to eliminate muscular tension. With feet on the floor, rest your arms easily in your lap or on the arms of the chair. Close your eyes and breathe in through your nose and out through your mouth, allowing your belly to be soft. Try to keep your mind blank; listen to your mind's voice say "soft" as you breathe in, and "relaxed" as you breathe out. If thoughts intrude, let them come and let them go.

A mantra is the second technique that can be used. It comes from Transcendental Meditation, which is of sub-continental Indian origin. A mantra is a special word we select for ourselves that frequently has a harmonious vibration internally and externally. It is a word that represents harmony with the universe, such as *one*, *peace*, or *love*. My personal mantra is "peace." I close my eyes and every time I exhale I see *peace*, either the word, or the letters, *p-e-a-c-e*, coming out of my mouth in smoke gradually floating up, forming the word. The mantra needs to fit our personal belief systems. Thus, some choose "Jesus," and others, "Relax." Although sleep is not part of this process, if time is not a premium, after ten to fifteen minutes many fall asleep and wake up extremely refreshed. During this period of relaxation the body rejuvenates to continue the day. When a stressful situation arises, I tell my patients to utter their mantra, or to go through the action of their mantra for a few seconds, and suddenly, like Pavlov's dogs, a programmed response relaxes the individual. You might remember that Pavlov rang a bell each time he fed a group of dogs. After several days of feeding, he rang the bell and the dogs would salivate even though there was no food. This is a conditioned response that happens in most animals, including humans. As the highest form of animal, we can learn from the others; dogs know about self-care, even if their masters do not.

Practicing a relaxation exercise, or a mantra, ten to forty-five minutes once or twice a day improves one's outlook, decreases anxiety, lowers blood pressure, and enables the whole body to work better. Plainly, these procedures are useful in the absence of illness, but they can also be applied to many medical diseases. Fertility, for instance, is enhanced, heart disease decreased, and pain syndromes improved, all along with the improvement of our general well-being.

The words *meditation* and *medicine* are derived from the same Sanskrit root word meaning "to take the measure of" and "to care for." Each of these definitions is apparent in our understanding of medicine: a potion to take, or a philosophy of care. Meditation accomplishes these, too, only quietly and internally. It takes measure of the moment and cares for the present. It is, by definition, the absence of neurosis, a condition of anxiety about what happened yesterday and the threat of tomorrow. In meditation, then, one experiences only the immediate; it requires being absolutely present. If thoughts come, let them go. This removes us from stress and fosters the body's own healing. Meditation is also powerful in preventing disease. As a result, it is beginning to come back into the mainstream medical field.

There are three kinds of meditation. The type I have outlined above is concentrated meditation. Here we concentrate on breathing and/or words. Prayers like, "Our Father who art in heaven...," or "Hail Mary," or "Hare Krishna, Hare Krishna..." are all examples of concentrated meditation. A second type is awareness, or mindful meditation. This involves becoming aware of thoughts, feelings, and sensations as they arise, and then consciously releasing them. A psychiatrist, for instance, might advise this for troubling emotions. The third type is expressive meditation, which is the oldest, least used, and, in some ways, the most potent. It includes dancing, shaking, twirling, drumming, and other physical expressions. Some of this occurs in religious settings such as davening (the orthodox Jewish practice of swaying forward and backward), chanting in a Catholic Mass, performing the repetitive tasks of Buddhism, raising the hands toward heaven in Christian charismatic services, speaking in tongues like Pentecostals, and dervish dancing. Singing, dancing, or cheering are secular examples of using one's body to express that which is internal.

High Five

With this method of meditation/relaxation, you inhale through the nose for a count of five, hold your breath in your lungs for a count of five, and then exhale the air through the nose for a count of five. When exhaling, the tip of the tongue should be touching the roof of the mouth, immediately in back of the front teeth. This is the yogic position that most enhances relaxation. I do this procedure five times a day; first thing in the morning, even before getting out of bed, and at the end of the day after I say my prayers, plus three times a day when I think about it. If a person does this exercise four times a day they will still be doing well. If it is hard to remember to do the exercises, simply do one before each meal. This will also relax you for the forthcoming meal, which will enhance your digestion. This is also a fringe benefit of praying before each meal.

There are other expressions of meditation in our everyday lives. Making love includes rhythmic and expressive body movements. Yoga and tai-chi are yet other examples of expressive meditation. The rhythmic moaning of people in pain is a natural example of meditation to relieve pain.

Music Heals

Listening to certain kinds of music, particularly Classical and Baroque, may be something you already enjoy doing, but did you know that it is a vehicle for relaxation and healing?

For a century, neuropsychologists have been working to improve the subconscious mind with methods such as neurolinguistic reprogramming (the unconscious formation of words), and subliminal messaging (speech below the audible threshold).

The melody, pitch, timing, and beat of such music as Pachebel's "Canon in D," and other Baroque classics and chants by the Benedictine Monks of Santo Domingo de Silos, can alter your state of being by quieting your mind and allowing you to enter its spiritual recesses.

Most scores of classical music range between 60 and 120 beats per minute. The resting heart beats approximately 50 to 60 times per minute, so it would appear that soothing scores in this range induce calm.

Another type of relaxation with music is "Binaural Beats," the term used for music with slightly different frequencies in each ear. The difference in these frequencies, or beats, elicits beneficial brain waves by releasing healthy neurotransmitters. So, in addition to drugs (antidepressants, energizers, and sleep aids), binaural music can help stress related or genetically endowed syndromes, such as insufficient sleep, chronic fatigue, fibromyalgia, dyslexia, and ADHD. Improved memory, learning, concentration, and creativity can be heightened with this technique.

By varying the difference of the frequencies in each individual ear, the brain wave frequency can be varied from 0 to 100 Hertz, and accordingly affect various parts of the brain. Neurotransmitters such as serotonin (which promotes relaxation and aids eating), noradrenalin (which promotes memory and physical performance), dopamine (which affects coordination and addictions), and acetycholine (which promotes memory with its various expressions) are increased or decreased. If the frequency was 410Hz in the left ear and 400Hz in the other, they would have a 10 beat difference, mimicking the Alpha state. But since the rhythm is the same, and there is such a small difference in pitch, the listener simply hears the music.

If this is performed while asleep, without the chatter of the external environment, the exchange can be enhanced fivefold. Stephen Halpern and Aeoliah (a Stage name) are both PhDs in music and psychology. They are both widely acknowledged as composers of music for health and healing. These pioneers of sound health brought the art and science of healing music into the field of complementary/integrative medicine and to the mainstream public through best-selling recordings. Unlike Binaural Music, one can listen without the need for ear buds.

This technique can help us to go from the deepest Delta wave (0 to 4 H), to the moderately deep Theta dream sleep (4 to 8 H), to the twilight Alpha (8 to 14 H), and the alert Beta (15 to 100 H) state. It is in the Delta state that super learning occurs and the youth-giving human growth hormone is released. There are applications for the iPhone for $1.99 that, with ear buds, can inspire you to creativity or mindful meditation and dream-filled sleep. Altered State and AmbiSci are two of the many apps offered. CDs are also available that can easily be put into a player with the same effect. (See LifeProgram.com.) For your mental and physical health, consider the music that heals.

EXERCISE MEDICINE

The following four types of exercise will keep you younger than your years—stretching, balancing, cardiovascular exercise, and strengthening.

Stretching

Stretching prevents injury to the muscle and its tendons and will keep you flexible. Formal exercises such as yoga, use of the exercise ball, or just plain yawning are healthful. Contrary to popular opinion, pulsing stretches should not be performed. Simply do gradual tightening until you experience mild discomfort of the muscle group, hold for a brief time, and then relax. This maneuver should be repeated three times. Hands to the sky, touching the toes, twisting the abdomen and chest on the pelvis from side to side, and pulling back the ankle to the buttock are some examples.

Balancing

Balancing is particularly helpful in older people. Good balance prevents falls and their potential for broken bones. Programs like tai chi and dancing are great, as is the big ball. After feeling confident sitting on the ball, try to recover after moving on the buttocks to a near-fall. Recently, the half ball has become inexpensively available to stand on. Simply standing on one foot for thirty seconds without holding on builds balance.

Cardiovascular Exercise

Cardiovascular endurance includes fast walking (until you experience slight shortness of breath), running up and down stairs, dancing, using a stationary bike, walking or jogging on a treadmill, running, jogging, or following along with an aerobic exercise DVD. Recently, HIIT— High Intensity Interval Training—has become popular. So I recommend 4 separate periods of peak effort ("bursts") for 60 seconds, such as running as fast as one can, or pushing the pedals as fast as possible. This builds up the mitochondria (the individual cellular motors) within the muscle fiber, enhancing the metabolism of fat, decreasing insulin resistance, and thus preventing cardiometabolic syndrome and diabetes. Moreover, this improves the most important muscle of the body, the heart.

Strengthening Exercise

Strengthening exercises build muscles and help turn fat into muscle. Weight lifting, resistance machines, and holding one's own weight against gravity (push-ups) are recommended. Fewer repetitions (reps) with heavy weights are suggested. Between eight and twelve reps with thirty seconds between sets is advised. The last rep should be so difficult that you could not do another one to "save your life." Bench and military presses, biceps curls, and shrugs are other examples of these. Three sets are suggested.

Home training is doable. Certainly it is easier to exercise in a gym and with a training partner who will hold you responsible if you do not show up. But if that is not possible, a workout can be done at home without any special equipment. Regularly perform squats and push-ups. Push-ups should be done by putting the toes and knees on the floor for women and the toes only on the floor for men, lying prone, and pushing up with your arms. Another type of exercise is a dip—place the back of your feet on one chair, your hands on the arms of another chair, and with your buttocks between the chairs, extend and flex your arms. Your abdominal muscles can be exercised by sit-ups: Lie on the floor with your toes under a piece of heavy furniture and sit up, touching your elbows to your knees.

Several variations of the sit-up are possible, such as touching your elbow to your opposite knee, or sitting only halfway up (crunch). Another exercise is to stand facing a wall and put your hands on it three feet or so from the floor, then push back. Recently, the Shake Weight has come on the market. In just six minutes a day, you can use this handy device to strengthen core and arm muscles.

These resistance exercises build muscle. Resistance exercises help more for weight loss than do cardio exercises. Another method of building healthy muscle is isometrics. Here you contract opposing muscle groups simultaneously and hold that tension using good posture as tight as you can for at least a minute. It is helpful to do this while looking into a mirror.

For every one pound of muscle an individual puts on, the body consumes an extra 100 calories to maintain and service that muscle. If you put on 5 pounds of muscle, you can have 500 free calories a day. This adds up to 3,500 calories a week, which is equivalent to one pound of weight loss! Jogging requires only a set of running shoes, and the "track" is just outside your front door. Once your ideal weight is obtained, keep on working out to maintain a healthy, better-looking body. Also burst extreme exercise decreases our telomere shortening thus extending not only our life, but our youth. More about telomeres below.

TELOMERES

Although many of us eat and maintain a healthy lifestyle to look and feel better, there is a superior reason for what we do: That is to *be better* and *live longer*. You can be productive and happy as a centenarian (someone living 100-plus years). How do you know how long and well they will live? Now there is a laboratory study for it, called telomere testing. Until the summer of 2010, the test was prohibitively expensive, but now many insurance companies pay for it or for less than $400 you can obtain your report card and intervene with their lifestyle to get a better and better score and either achieve their goal or come very close to it.

Telomeres are sections of DNA at the end of each chromosome whose primary function is to prevent chromosomal "fraying" when a cell replicates. As a cell ages, its telomeres become shorter. How much shorter is governed by genetic factors and environmental stressors. Eventually, the telomeres become too short to allow cell replication, the cell stops dividing, and ultimately dies, which is a normal biological process. The more of our cells die, the older and frailer we become until we ourselves die—in that all our reserves are gone and we succumb to disease or just old age. A telomere test can determine the length of a patient's telomeres in relation to their chronological age. The Patient Telomere Score is calculated based on the telomere length on the patient's white blood cells (T-lymphocytes). This is then compared to the average telomere length on lymphocytes from a sample of the American population in the same age range. The higher the telomere score, the "younger" the cells and the longer and better that person will live. The test can be repeated annually, and the patient can then work harder or intervene in other ways to enhance their score and their life.

Diet plays a large role in telomere length. The best but the most difficult form of diet is caloric restriction to the point of just sustenance, a step away from starvation. Far easier and almost as good is eating correctly for your Apo-E type, going easy on meat, eating whole nutrient-dense foods, as raw as possible, consuming Omega 3s, and staying away from grains and processed foods. According to a study in the January 20, 2010, issue of *JAMA*, increased telomere and survival rates occurred among individuals with high dietary intake of marine Omega 3 fatty acids and established cardiovascular disease. In this five-year study, the researchers found that individuals with the lowest DHA+EPA experienced the most rapid rate of telomere shortening, whereas those in the highest had the slowest rate of shortening. Higher levels of DHA+EPA were associated with less telomere shortening before and after sequential adjustment for established risk factors and potential confounders. For each 1-standard deviation increase in red cell Omega 3 levels, there was a 32 percent reduction in the odds of telomere shortening! Both the micronutrient and the Omega 3 levels tests are available at some labs and physicians' offices and is performed by Spectracell Laboratories.

Minimizing emotional (psychological) and physiological (infectious, traumatic, or surgical) stress will keep your telomeres longer and you healthier. Additionally, increasing antioxidants slows telomere shortening. Physical exercise with adequate antioxidants will also give longer telomeres. Common sense dictates that decreasing cardiovascular risk factors (lipids, homocysteine, blood pressure, Hs-C reactive protein, glucose, etc.) and correcting micronutrient deficencies (vitamins, minerals, and glutathione) will preserve the telomere length. Periodically getting rid of our poison buildup by colonic and liver cleanses and from the skin by sweating (artificially by sauna or by heavy exercise) and minimizing the toxins in our water, air, and food will go a long way in keeping our telomeres longer. Keeping our hormones (thyroid, sex, and adrenal) in balance and not getting sick also keeps our telomeres longer. To not get sick means keeping our immune system healthy to include the consumption of pre- and probiotics such as hi-maize-amylose-resistant cornstarch laced with *Lactobacillus rhamnosus* (PL60) and other Bacteroidetes species. Surgery should be only for lifesaving problems and not for elective procedures since the operation and the anesthesia shortens the telomers. Staying out of harm's way for bodily damage in our daily pursuits, such as not overindulging in alcohol and dangerous sports and occupations, will keep our telomeres and our lives longer.

Bypassing Bypass

Helping the heart to grow new blood vessels is the biological way to bypass clogged coronary arteries. The *unnatural* method is the common procedures of angioplasty, with or without stents, and bypass arterial surgery. These revascularization measures are invasive, costly, potentially painful, frequently temporary, and *dangerous*. Double blind studies compared to "Optimum Medical Therapy" show minimal advantage for these invasive procedures, which can cause morbidity and mortality. In over 5,000 studies exercise has shown to benefit coronary artery disease and prevent heart attacks. One way extreme exercise helps is to nudge collateral dormant vessels to develop and prosper. These tiny blood vessels in the proximity of the obstructed artery have been sitting there since birth; they can potentially elongate and widen to circumvent the blocked artery.

Intense exercise generates a host of chemical and physical signals both locally in the heart and systemically throughout the body. It is postulated that AGF (angiogenesis growth factor) stimulates the progressive expansion of these embryonic arteries to reroute the blood flow around the blocked vessels. Such a natural bypass keeps the heart muscle well supplied with oxygen-rich blood as much as the invasive counterparts of angioplasty/stent and surgery. But to do this the individual must go to the limit of endurance. Many doctors are hesitant to have their patients push themselves physically, fearing they may do even more heart damage. While I was in medical school in 1962, a study published by Vojin Smodaka, a cardiologist in Valley Forge Medical Center, got my attention. In those days physicians would treat their patients with bed rest for two weeks, then limited physical activity for the rest of their lives. He showed that extreme exercise in the form of bursts (HIIT—High Intensity Interval Training) was not only safe, but reconditioned the heart. Nowadays most doctors do advise some excerise.

After doing a stress exercise treadmill test on the patient, observing for heart strength, blood pressure, and electrical activity, I advise patients to do aggressive aerobic exercise. This should be in the form that suits the person best. Occasionally it is done by swimming, but mostly it is done on a treadmill (or better, outside running), stationary bike, elliptical machine, or the stair stepper. They do alternatively bursts of intense activity with periods of gentler movement. For example, after gradually working up to it on a treadmill, they pace themselves at four miles an hour and every three minutes go to eight mph for *one minute*. If they can do that without having too much shortness of breath (dyspnea) or chest discomfort, they increase the speed another 0.2 miles per hour and so on. The more dyspnea, or mild chest pain, they have, the more AGF is stimulated and the better the collaterals grow. As a fringe benefit of this exercise, fat decreases, the patient feels better physically and mentally, and their blood sugar and lipids improve.

Let Your Food Be Your Medicine

Hipocrates said, "Let food be your medicine, and medicine your food." In other words, put the "farm" in "pharmacology." Though this may sound glib, it is, pragmatically, correct. In addition to nutritional foods, which will be discussed in greater detail later, there are many medicinal herbs that can be included in our diets. Ginger for nausea, garlic for lowering blood pressure, chamomile for relaxation, and black cohosh for menopausal symptoms are just a few examples. Each food has certain molecular structures that stimulate various receptors in the intestine and other tissues when delivered in the bloodstream. Food allergies also affect total health. Some people are acutely allergic to foods like shellfish or peanuts, which can cause immediate life-threatening reactions such as restricted airways or even anaphylactic shock. Most food allergies, however, are subtle. Gluten intolerance, for example, can cause acne and migraines.

Using specialized laboratories, I have have conducted food tests with very good results. For example, some individuals had no "allergic" problem eating wheat, but when they stopped eating gluten they felt better, slept more soundly, and had less respiratory illness. In the past we have diagnosed food sensitivities through elimination diets, but now we have blood tests that target specific food intolerance.

Changing your diet accordingly can make significant differences in diseases such as chronic fatigue syndrome, irritable bowel disease, seizure disorders, and ADHD. In migraine studies, for example, 92 percent of the individuals tested had noticeably fewer headaches simply by removing from their diets foods to which they were sensitive, such as coffee, chocolate, lunchmeat, sharp cheeses, and wine. These food intolerances can be easily identified, making medicinal eating another aspect of self-care.

What Should We Eat?

There is no best diet, but there is fundamental nutrition. There is an ideal diet for that individual for that given time depending on their genes, biology, age, and environment. Having an understanding of this new nutrition will enable a person to choose the correct foods for both health and longevity. The following information should help you make the right choices. The underpinnings of our food and drink should be for what we were genetically adapted. However, there are rarely two of us who are exactly alike, either in how we look in our faces or how we act metabolically. Our genes have been in existence since the very beginning of life on earth, but our current chromosomes have been here for 2.4 million years and have sustained man as a species for the last two hundred thousand years. But eating habits, desire, and in particular food availability determined what consumption in Homosapiens was best for theirs and now our health and fitness. This timeline represents 99 percent of our evolutionary history. It is only in the last 25 thousand years that we evolved from gatherers, pickers, fishers, pluckers, and ghouls* to hunters. As a species, we hunted small game and fish with our hands and our cunning for eons, but with the advent of tools like nets, spears, and clubs, big game became obtainable for hunting groups for 15 thousand years. In only the last 10 thousand years agriculture and later animal husbandry naturally developed. Most importantly in the dawn of the Industrial Revolution, refined foods became available to the masses. But our metabolic machinery was not prepared for this. We are still in the state of evolution and may never be prepared for the junk we consume in the name of food!

No one would argue that an infant needs a different diet from an adult, or that a Type 1 diabetic needs a dissimilar diet from a "healthy" individual, or an elderly person another fare than a younger. But the fact that a female diet needs to be different from a male's may be a stretch for some. In the broader sense, scientists and pseudo-scientists have organized special diets for metabolic types based on blood type, body shapes (apples versus pears), personalities, or even anthropomorphic measurements such as arm span and variations of tooth anatomy. We are now able to do an insurance-paid genetic test (offered by Genalix) that an under-the-tongue swab can determine the specific metabolism of food and drugs. Here are some basic truths for human food consumption and life and a few more for a healthy existence:

- The human body (and most mammals) has a given requirement for protein and fat, but *none* for carbohydrate other than disposable energy.

*Ghoul: Early man ate bone marrow and brains from carrion and at times of other humans in that he had rock tools and the knowledge to open bones.

- Carbohydrate is a fuel that is converted to glucose for immediate usage or is made and stored in the liver as animal starch, or glycogen.

- Micronutrients (vitamins, macro-minerals, trace minerals) are needed in adequate amounts for proper metabolism.

- Essential fatty acids are necessary for both for the structure and function of the organism.

- Essential amino acids are also obligatory for the formation and working of the living being.

- Glyconutrients (on cell walls for inner communication) from sugars can be internally produced from non-carbohydrate foodstuffs.

- Enough water is required to maintain the shape and flow of our life form.

- Fiber is needed to give substance to the food in our alimentary tract to properly propel it forward and to feed our gut flora.

- Bacteria (probiotic) and its food (prebiotic), which is soluble fiber, are required to complete our digestion and to produce micronutrients such as Vitamin B12.

Gluten Sensitivity

Celiac disease is vastly underdiagnosed. It takes an average of eleven years between the first appearances of bowel symptoms to its diagnosis. To add insult to injury, many times it is silent in the intestine and where extra-intestinal problems occur. The most common significant allergen known to civilized man is gluten, a protein frequently found in wheat. As many as 10 percent of us are sensitive to it. Gluten is also found in rye, spelt, triticale, and kamut. Although not all doctors agree, it may also be found in dark beans, oats, and peanuts. Non-gluten cereals are rice, tapioca, buckwheat, flaxseed, millet, teff, and quinoa (*keen-wa*). It is not found in vegetables and meat. Gluten is used in 90 percent of all protein-fortified products. When this foreign protein is ingested, it attacks the intestine, causing inflammation and poor absorption of nutrients. To add insult to injury, another harmful mechanism comes into play. Zonulin is a protein in the intestinal wall that regulates the absorption of nutrients. Its job is to open and close spaces between tightly-packed cells that line the small intestine, letting vital nutrients in, and keeping destructive proteins, like gluten, out. Too much zonulin such as in folks who have gluten intolerance and jams the space the open. With this come bits and pieces of larger food protein that also form antibodies in that it is foreign to our bodies. This plays even more havoc with our tissues causing reaction in our organs. Therefore Gluten and other antigens cause antibodies destroying some of our other tissues.

This genetic malady is termed celiac disease when it involves the intestine so that malabsorption occurs. But that is only part of the problem. The age of onset can be anywhere from infancy to senility. Children with celiac disease develop neurological symptoms, short stature, and anemia. In adults, the following symptoms occur: skin rashes, particularly dermatitis herpetiformis; osteoporosis; anemia; infertility; irritable bowel syndrome; GERD; neurological symptoms; autoimmune diseases such as low thyroid (Hashimoto's disease); arthritis; and vitiligo. Lymphoma and other cancers are more common in folks who have sensitivity to gluten and still consume it.

Gluten intolerance is frequently caused by some preceding damage to the lining of the intestines from toxic exposures, infections, or medications. Gluten intolerance, like true celiac disease, is treated by avoiding gluten. I tell people with this intolerance to stay away from *BROWS*: where *B* stands for Barley and Beans (green), *R* for Rye, *O* for Oats, *W* for Wheat, and *S* for Spelt. The three criteria for true celiac disease are a genetic predisposition, the consumption of gluten, and a triggering event, which could be physical or emotional. With the loss of the integrity of the intestinal lining, the small intestine fails to absorb the micronutrients, which affects all tissues of the body. Rarely are the typical symptoms related to just the gastrointestinal tract with abdominal pain and distention, diarrhea, and weight loss.

We have evolved as cereal-less Homo sapiens for almost 500,000 years. The first wheat was accidently noted and occasionally gathered about 8,000 BC. The first wheat farmers came to be in England about 5,500 years ago. So we as a species went from great hunters to canaries in only 10,000 years! Science knows it takes much longer to change our genes to adapt to the gluten protein. Frequently, our bodies still see gluten as a foreigner rather than a "non-intruder." There was no wheat in the Garden of Eden. Adam and Eve and their myriad of descendants were never meant to eat this "food."

At least a third of gluten-intolerent people have lactose problems. The consumption of pizza, of which the dough is an extremely potent reactant, along with the cheese can cause acute symptoms within twenty minutes.

Discovered in Poland in 1953, but not known to the Western world until popularized by the English expert James Braly, MD, many celiacs have a foreshortened fifth finger (Braly's sign). This is to say that the end of the pinkie is shorter than the last joint of the ring finger.

To document the diagnosis, many doctors do a few blood studies that are only positive if the patient has terrible bowel disease when the blood is drawn and is still consuming gluten.[1] For now, most doctors feel there is no cure for gluten intolerance and the best way to alleviate symptoms is to stay away from food containing gluten. However, there is at least one naturopath who champions a gluten "cure" with the use of homeopathics and supplements for just one month. Very soon there will be a product (Larazotide Acetate) on the market that will allow a gluten intolerant to ingest some gluten without much problem.

NICOTINE

Nicotine in tobacco has brought illness and death to millions of people. Yet nicotine in its pure form has the potential to be a valuable pharmaceutical agent. Nicotine specifically binds to the cholinergic nicotinic gating site on cationic ion channels in receptors throughout the body. This action stimulates the release of a variety of neurotransmitters, especially catecholamines and serotonin in the brain. This is why it has shown to improve memory in general, and in particular in Alzheimer's patients. Also, when chronically taken, nicotine may result in positive reinforcement, negative reinforcement, reduction in body weight, enhancement of performance, and protection against Parkinson's disease, Tourette's syndrome, ulcerative colitis, and sleep apnea. The reliability of these effects varies greatly, but they justify the search for more therapeutic applications for this very interesting compound.

Dr. C. S. Myers from the clinical pharmacology and therapeutics branch of the National Institute on Drug Abuse, of NIH, published a double-blind study showing the benefits of nicotine. The discovery of the role of nicotinic receptors in attention and memory has led to the testing of nicotinic analogs as cognitive-enhancing agents in patient populations. Empirical information about nicotine's ability to enhance elements of attention and memory in normal individuals might guide development of therapeutic uses of nicotine in cognitively impaired populations. These results, based on a nicotine nasal spray, indicates a dose-related enhancement, particularly among women. This provides additional proof that nicotine improves attentional and computational abilities in non-deprived smokers and may be helpful in the treatment of Alzheimer's.

VINPOCETINE

A chemical that is related to nicotine is vinpocetine, an alkaloid from Vinca minor (periwinkle). It was introduced thirty-two years ago in Hungary for the treatment of vascular dementia—a disorder resulting from insufficient blood flow to the brain tissue. Prescriptive vinpocetine has gained popularity as a European "smart drug." Recently it has become available in the United States because of the lack of FDA supervision, so it is now considered a supplement. It is a promising neuroprotective supplement and cognitive booster. It is interesting that vinpocetine has a similar mechanism of action as that of Viagra. Both are known to be effective phosphodiesterase inhibitors. That is, they work to enhance blood flow by inhibiting an enzyme in the phosphodiesterase family. Not surprisingly, the main benefit of vinpocetine is an improvement in cerebral blood flow. More blood reaching the brain cells means better oxygenation, nutrition, and waste removal—all of which adds up to more youthful brain function.

Vinpocetine has also been found to improve the transport of glucose (both uptake and release) across the blood-brain barrier. Low cellular energy production is perhaps the primary factor underlying all aging-related brain degeneration. In addition, vinpocetine has been shown to increase the firing rate of certain types of noradrenergic neurons, which could explain one mechanism of its action as a cognitive booster. The enhancement of blood flow and energy production means that vinpocetine is particularly recommended for people whose cognitive dysfunction stems chiefly from insufficient blood flow to the brain. Vinpocetine also shows promise in helping prevent damage to vision, especially dry macular degeneration. Vinpocetine likewise appears to improve blood flow to the inner ear, thus protecting hearing. Interestingly, vinpocetine has also been found to counteract motion sickness. It can also partly protect against the damage resulting from excess glutamate and other excitotoxins.

A new neuroprotective property of vinpocetine has just been discovered. It can lower the production of inflammatory cytokines. Together with other phosphodiesterase inhibitors, vinpocetine has been shown to lower the production by the microglia of a major inflammatory compound known as tumor necrosis factor-alpha (TNF-alpha). Some alternative clinicians believe that if we could truly control inflammation, we could prevent Alzheimer's disease. This view is based on the proven effectiveness of anti-inflammatories, such as ibuprofen, in lowering the risk of Alzheimer's disease. The problem with commonly used pharmaceutical anti-inflammatories is their side effects. Vinpocetine and other natural anti-inflamma-tories (fish oil, vitamin E, estrogens, and many antioxidants, including bilberry extract and green tea catechins) appear to be a nontoxic alternative.

Vinpocetine is an alkaloid, in the same family as caffeine and nicotine, both known to be very effective cognitive enhancers. Nicotine increases the release of acetylcholine and dopamine, and it improves both short-term recall and long-term potentiation. But while caffeine and nicotine each have well-known drawbacks, vinpocetine appears to be safe and non-addictive. It would not be surprising if vinpocetine shared nicotine's protective benefits against Alzheimer's and Parkinson's disease, without the problem of addiction.

An interesting side benefit of vinpocetine is that it has also been found to protect against both gastric and cerebral damage induced by alcohol, against kidney problems caused by renal vasoconstriction, and against hepatic damage caused by the hepatitis B. It is supplied in 1, 5, and 10 mg tablets. I usually recommend 10 mg twice a day, then increase to 30 and even 40 mg. There are no interactions with other drugs.

Is Apo-E Right for Me?

Apolipoprotein E (Apo-E), a blood test to predict premature cardiovascular and/or Alzheimer's disease, was prohibitively expensive until June 2010. At that time, the Athrotec Corporation and later Spectrocell reduced the price to about thirty dollars as an add-on study. It is paid for by most insurance companies.

Each of us is given two copies (allels) of Apo-E at birth, and they remain the same throughout life. Therefore, if you take the test once, you never have to take it again. There is no Apo-E e1. We have one *each* of 2, 3, and 4. A person can have e2/23 or e2/e4 or double of each, such as e4/e4. Those with Apo-E e2/e2 alleles are at a higher risk of premature vascular disease, although some people will never develop the disease, depending on their lifestyle. Likewise, they may have the disease but not have e2/e2 alleles, because it is only one of the factors involved.

Our genes cannot change, but they can be modified by our diet, exercise, and medications. Apo-E genotyping provides us with additional information, and if symptoms are present, learning your alleles can help confirm Type 3 hyperlipoproteinemia, which has chylomicron (fat/triglyceride globules) remnants and very low density lipoprotein (VLDL) particles that should be rapidly removed from the circulation by the liver. Apolipoprotein-E, the main component of the chyhlomicron and VLDL, binds to a specific receptor on liver cells for disposal. So Apo-E is essential for the normal metabolism of triglycerides and cholesterol.

In addition to predicting age of death, Apo-E helps us determine if we will get Alzheimer's before we die. This is the most common form of dementia. This incurable, degenerative, and terminal disease was first described by German psychiatrist and neuropathologist Alois Alzheimer in 1906 and was named after him. Generally it is diagnosed in people over sixty-five years of age, although the less prevalent early-onset Alzheimer's can occur much earlier. In 2010, there were 30.6 million sufferers worldwide. Alzheimer's is predicted to affect one in eighty-five people globally by 2050. The Apo-E test will go a long way toward predicting it so that, should you have the alleles for it, you can do things now to prolong its onset and even prevent it!

The earliest observable symptoms of Alzheimer's disease are often mistaken for "age-related" concerns, or manifestations of stress. In the early stages, the commonly recognized symptom is an inability to acquire new memories, such as difficulty in recalling recently observed facts. As the disease advances, symptoms begin to include confusion, irritability and aggression, mood swings, language breakdown, long-term memory loss, and the general withdrawal of the sufferer as their senses decline. Gradually, body functions are lost, ultimately leading to death. Individual prognosis is difficult to assess, as the duration of the disease varies. Alzheimer's disease develops for an indeterminate period of time before becoming fully apparent, and it can progress undiagnosed for years. The mean life expectancy following diagnosis is approximately seven years. Fewer than 3 percent of individuals live more than fourteen years after diagnosis. When Alzheimer's is suspected, the diagnosis is usually confirmed with behavioral assessments and cognitive tests, such as an MMSE or a CDR. I often order an MRI to look at the hippocampel volume, and if I am in real doubt, I order a PET scan with a PIB contrast.

Over 60 percent of those who have late onset Alzheimer's have paired Apo-E e4 alleles (e4/e4). The E4 variant is the largest known genetic risk factor for late-onset Alzheimer's disease in a variety of ethnic groups. Caucasian and Japanese carriers of two E4 alleles have *ten times* the risk of developing Alzheimer's by seventy-five years of age, as compared to those the pair of E4 alleles.

Research suggests an interaction with amyloid. Alzheimer's is characterized by plaques consisting of amyloid. Apo-E enhances proteolytic breakdown of this peptide, both within and between cells. S Apo-E 4 is not as efficient as others at catalyzing these reactions resulting in increased vulnerability to Alzheimer's in individuals with this gene variation. Among Apo-E4 carriers, another gene, GAB-2 is thought to further influence the risk of getting Alzheimer's. However, the relationship does not appear as strong as E4, since in the Japanese, GAB-2 is not a risk factor. There is also evidence that Apo-E 2 allele may serve a protective role in preventing Alzheimer's and maybe heart disease. Thus, the genotype most at risk for developing Alzheimer's and cardiovascular disease at an earlier age is Apo-E 4/4. The Apo-E 3/4 genotype is at increased risk, though not to the degree that those with 4/4 are. The genotyupe Apo-E 3/3 is considered at normal risk for these, and the genotype e2/e3 is considered at a less risk. Interestingly, People with both a copy of the Apo-E 2/4, are at ordinary risk, just as those with the genotype Apo-E 3/3. Apo E4s do not respond well to the statins, very heavy exercise, and any fat other than DHA and Cocconut Oil.

Keys to Longevity

Hunza is located in the far northeast of Pakistan, in a remote valley some 200 miles long but only one mile wide. It is situated at an elevation of 8,500 feet and is completely enclosed by mountain peaks to include the Himalayans. The fabled brigadoon is said to have been inspired by Hunza. The inhabitants, Hunzakuts, have the reputation of being the longest lived people in the world. They eat fresh, mostly raw fruits and vegetables and little meat. Of course, there are no pesticides or preservatives in them. However, it is generally accepted that the water the Hunzas drink plays a major role in their great health and longevity. This water comes from the melting of the glaciers from the nearby mountains. These glaciers are hundreds of thousand years old and grind the mountainous rock into extremely fine particles. In turn, the fine particles of rock are suspended in this water and is called glacial milk because of its cloudy appearance by being so loaded with these minerals. Coming from glacial mountain streams and waterfalls, this water carries a negative charge or negative ions and is called "living water." This results in the water having an oxygen-reduction potential and acts as an antioxidant in the body with the ability to neutralize free radicals. Also the negative charge makes minerals easily absorbable. Their crops are also irrigated with this colloidal alkalizing mineral water and thus unlike Western soils, Hunza soils are not depleted of minerals.

This living water can almost be duplicated today by Kangen, which is a Japanese word best translated into English as "Return to Original," which means several things when used to describe water. It is alkaline, ionized, anti-oxidant electron rich, restructured, micro clustered, active hydrogen saturated, and oxidation reduced. Water is first purified, then given an electrical charge to recreate electron rich water. This electrolysis process using a platinum catalyst on a titanium base is first put through a special charcoal filter. It contains the essential minerals, and the pH can be set from 2.5 to 11.5, but for drinking purposes 8.5 is the best.

The very alkaline water (pH-11.5) is used in place of damaging chemicals for cleaning and disinfecting around the home, especially the bathroom and kitchen. It is an emulsifier and used plain is a fantastic detergent to get the pesticides off fruits and vegetables, clear greasy grime, and even unclog drains. Topically, it can be used as a poultice on inflamed skin. On the other side of the pH, the acid (2.5) is a powerful disinfectant for bacteria, yeast, and viruses.

In addition to the Hunza, there are three other other long-lived healthy people on our planet. Dan Buettner published in the *National Geographic*, and later in his book, *The Blue Zones*, details his studies of Sardinia, Okinawa, and a group of Seventh-Day Adventists in Loma Linda, California.

Sardinia, a small island in the Mediterranean, has the highest longevity in all of Europe. There, a man is 160 times more likely to live to be 100, compared to Germany. These people originally came from the Basque area of Spain, and migrated to this small island 16,000 years ago. First the Phoenicians, then the Roman invaders pushed them into the mountains with their harsh climate. The men were shepherds, spending as much as three months in near isolation while the sheep grazed the mountain meadows. The women worked at home raising the children, taking care of finances, and producing dairy products from sheep's milk. They did the worrying and the men did the physical work. Their food was mostly dairy loaded with CLA (conjugated linoleic acid) from the mountainside grass. The people drank a strong, extremely dark wine with meals and ate special, whole grain bread (musica). Occasionally, the table would be graced with fish from the sea (sardines) and, rarely, mutton as a garnish. Lifestyle and diet changes after World War II resulted in obesity rising from 1 percent of the population to 35 percent, while life expectancy declined 25 percent.

The Seventh-Day Adventists, of which there are 12 million, have been studied by the National Institute of Health over the last four decades. They consume a biblical diet (see Genesis 1:29), do not smoke or drink, routinely exercise, zealously go to church, take the Sabbath off, and consume a plant-based diet with emphasis on nuts. A recently published study shows that those who were strict in their religious observations lived, on average, 87 years for males and 88.5 years for women. Those who were less strict in their observance, lived an average of ten years less and had many more disabilities in their last decade of life.

Older Okinawans have the longest lifespan without disability in the world, with only one-fifth the rate of breast and colon cancer and one-sixth the incidence of cardiovascular disease compared to the United States. The indigenous people are remotely and racially distinct from the Japanese and live in a mountainous, primitive island environment. Their food consists of meat only once a year on New Year's Day, when they butcher the family pig. They occasionally eat seafood, lots of tofu, nuts, and sweet potatoes. They use ginger and tumeric (curcumin) generously as condiments.

Family values are high. They have great respect for their elders, whom they venerate during life and beyond. The older the individuals, the more wisdom and honor they are believed to have. Children are encouraged to form a small core group called "moyai." These groups consist of four to six childhood friends of the same sex who bond in their youth and maintain a close relationship throughout life. Since these people rarely move, this clique remains physically, socially, and spiritually together for a lifetime, getting together at least weekly. They share both their fortunes and misfortunes. Chairs are a rarity; sitting and sleeping on the floor is the rule. This translates to forced exercise by getting up many times a day. Perhaps most importantly, the inhabitants encourage a life goal, or *"ike gai,"* which is their reason to get up in the morning. In eating, they practice *"hara hachi bu,"* which is eating only until the belly is 80 percent full. After World War II, Americanization came to the islands, with all of its good and bad practices. Okinawa is a protectorate of the United States. Early on, they were given K-rations, which contained canned ham products, and now they have the world's highest per capita consumption of Spam. They are now also the largest consumers of fast foods in the world, thanks to our influence.

Now those inhabitants who are less than fifty years old have the highest numbers of obesity of any people on earth, despite the fact that those over seventy have the highest incidence of centenarians in the world.

When one synthesizes the beliefs and practices of the Seventh-Day Adventists, the Sardinians, and the Okinawans, seven facts can be distilled: 1. Don't smoke; 2. Get moderate daily exercise; 3. Eat mostly a plant-based diet; 4. Have a sense of purpose, ("*ike gai*"); 5. Invest your time and energy in family and community; 6. "*Hara hachi bu*": Eat only to 80 percent fullness and leave the table slightly hungry; 7. Take your time at meals, chew well, and celebrate your food; 8, Believe in a higher power; 9. Be optimistic; 10. Drink a little wine.

Disease As a Wakeup Call

We all hope to stay healthy physically, psychologically, and financially. Being gainfully employed can serve each of these desires. It's not just about making money for money's sake, or to put food on the table, for the small and large luxuries in life, or for financial security in our old age, but it should be about fulfilling our purpose on this earth. Disease can interrupt our goals, but illness can also be a great teacher. Illness certainly gets our attention. Surviving a heart attack because of stress-induced hypertension and high cholesterol is a stimulus for change.

Having a different attitude toward your job and transforming your values to emphasize your family and your spiritual health, can make a large difference in the quality and quantity of your life. This does not mean that we always cause our own sickness, but it does mean that if we have a disease, we can look at it as an opportunity for transformation. It may be a sign that we are out of balance; the particular disease may give us a clue to the imbalance. Furthermore, if we look at disease as nothing more than a misfortune, we will only see ourselves as victims. If we instead look at it as an opportunity to learn and grow, then we become students of our own lives with self-directed goals for productivity and satisfaction. In any condition of health or illness, we need to validate our worth to give us a sense of fulfillment.

True fulfillment has a deeper source than financial gain; heaven itself may be reflected in our enjoyment of our work. Though it might sound lofty or idealistic, we need to perceive a calling beyond the noisy demands of daily life, something that echoes within us saying, "This is the work I am meant to do; it is my life's work." If we do not pursue this, we are bound to languish mentally, spiritually, and physically. Disease may be caused by neglecting our life's purpose. We are profoundly blessed if our avocation can be our vocation. This does not apply only to professionals or craftsmen, either. Men and women who cultivate their heartfelt desires by nurturing families, relationships, careers, or any other conviction will find the same satisfaction in life. This is a process of development and of understanding who we are, what we are meant to be, and what we are doing on this planet. It is not necessarily excitement or momentary exhilaration we should seek, but *contentment*. This sort of indulgence improves our lives and inspires those around us. We, as physicians, should remind our patients of this philosophy; too often the stresses of illness nearly obliterate it. So, find a physician who is sensitive to these concerns, or teach your favorite doctor to be.

A Healthy Marriage, A Healthy Life

Married couples live longer than those who are unmarried and live together, or those who live alone. Marriage is associ-

Rules of Engagement and Endearment

Based on the movie *"Fireproof"* and the book *"The Love Dare"*

Speak with your spouse at a peaceful time about these.

1. We wil never mention divorce.

2. We will not bring up old, unrelated items from the past.

3. We will never fight in public or in front of our chldren.

4. We will call a "time out" if conflict escalates to a damaging level.

5. We will never touch or talk to one another in a harmful and abusive way.

6. We will never go to bed angry with one another.

ated with greater health, self-esteem, happiness, and satisfaction. This is true for both good and bad marriages, but obviously with good marriages it is even more so. Each of us is an individual with our own desires, emotions, and ways of doing things. Going through the motions of a happy marriage is a good way to create a happy marriage—no matter how bad yours might seem at the time.

The Proper Care and Feeding of Marriage, by Dr. Laura Schlesinger, is a marriage bible in which she states: "Treat your spouse as if you love them with your last breath, no matter how contrary that might feel at that moment. Think hard every day about how you can make your spouse's life worth living and be the person you would want to love, hug, come home to, and sacrifice for."

The ingredients of a good marriage are approval, attention, affection, and sex. These commitments were made in your marriage vows. The Lord has given you sensuality to be used not only frequently but appropriately. See yourselves as a team and not enemies or competitors. Do not let toxic thoughts bring you down. Is it not better to be loved than to be right? Early love is when you love the way another person makes you feel, but mature love is when you love the person as he or she is. No one is responsible for our happiness but us, and we don't have control over the other person, only ourselves. With this in mind, and knowing we can't force anyone to change, we can change ourselves. When you can enjoy loving and being loved, needing and being needed, changing your mind-set is a small price to pay.

Puppy love causes the release of various hormones, particularly phenylethylalanine, which gives you the *heartfelt* desire to be with your mate in an early stage of a relationship. After months or years, that feeling fades. But if you honor your commitment to marriage and keep doing the right things, these feelings are replaced with something far deeper and precious. Give, give, and give some more. Soon, your spouse will do the same. It should be "we" and not "me," and the whole (the family) is greater than the sum of its parts. Don't keep score of what your spouse has done. Marriage is not about equal duty; it's about equal commitment. If you change your thinking about marriage and do it correctly, you'll get the only respect that matters—self-respect—and so will your spouse.

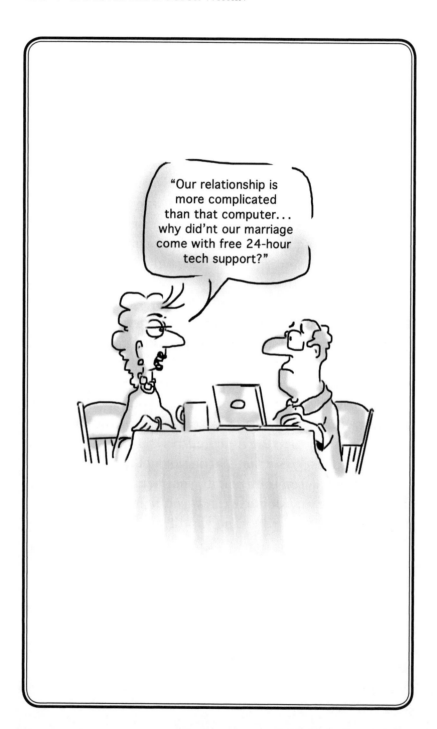

3

Food

Basics

Food is any organic substance used as a fuel to energize and build our living tissue. Our metabolism converts some of it to basic building-blocks that are as fundamental to our constitution as our genes. In fact, eating and drinking wisely allows us to overrule our genes. We are one of the few animals on earth that can do this.

Food can be divided into *macronutrients*, of which there are three: fats, proteins, and carbohydrates; and *micronutrients*, of which there are over 2,500. These contribute to our energy and structure. If taken in the proper proportions, we can obtain the ideal health, shape, and weight for our genes (or jeans, if you prefer). The proportion of each has been argued vigorously by nutritionists, physicians, and scientists for hundreds of years. According to the American Heart Association, fat was supposed to be the villain, and to some of my colleagues it still is. I, like many other experts, feel it is not the fat but the carbs, particularly crapohydrates (a glycemic index greater than 50), which make us unhealthily fat! If we go back to our biology and eat and work like a caveman, we can achieve a lean, strong healthy body and soul. To this I would add that the sources of the macronutrients should correspond to our blood type and, if possible, body type; it must also accommodate our food intolerances. This personalized amalgamation of diets helps us feel better, discourages weight gain, decreases allergies, and gives us more energy. The less prepared the food and the less cooked, the better. Raw vegetables contain enzymes easily destroyed in cooking.

Unfortunately, overeating has been built into our genetic code. Because of frequent famines and other conditions of scarcity, even after the development of agriculture, humans learned to overeat whenever possible. Even our gut bacteria are thrifty and can make simple sugars out of fiber. It was survival not of the fittest, but of the fattest. Now, after years of plenty, being overweight has reached epidemic proportions.

Our genes are of ancient origin—they are as much as two million years old. Research has shown that chimpanzees are only 1.6 percent different from us, genetically. The collective human genome has changed only minimally since modern Homo sapiens became widespread about thirty-five thousand years ago. We are classified as omnivores, and though we eat flesh, or meat, like carnivores, our metabolism is more like that of herbivores. Carnivores have claws, while herbivores have hands or hoofs. The teeth of a carnivore are sharp, but the teeth of an herbivore are mainly flat for grinding. The intestinal tract is short in a carnivore, but the human intestine is twenty-six feet long. A carnivore cools its body by panting; an herbivore sweats. The biggest difference, depending on our genetic makeup, is how food is metabolized and what micronutrients we need. Carnivores manufacture their own vitamin C, and like herbivores, we must obtain it from our diet. Furthermore, when we eat like carnivores we are more likely to elevate certain chemicals like uric acid and lipids in our bodies to dangerous levels which causes gout, and cardiovascular disease.

Fish- and Plant-Based Nutrients for Health

For years scientists have told us that eating plants is healthier than eating meats, but since the twenty-five-year China Study was published in 2002, and in the September 2010 *NEJM*, in which the *Nurses Health Study* has shown no doubt about the fact that meats (bovine, sheep, pork, goat) should be eaten in moderation or not at all, depending on one's genetics, particularly those Apo-E4s which requires no fat. Poultry and principally fish are good sources of protein. When eating the bulk of your food, which should be vegetables, *it should be the leaves, flower, and stems rather than the roots and fruits* that should be consumed. Nutrient density is an important concept in dietary recommendations. Not merely vitamins and minerals, but adequate consumption of phytochemicals is essential for proper functioning of the immune system and to enable our body's detoxification and cellular repair mechanisms that protect us from gaining fat and the consequences of chronic disease. To guide people toward the most nutrient-dense foods, a scoring system called ANDI (Aggregate Nutrient Density Index), or *HANDY ANDI*, which ranks foods based on their ratio of nutrients to calories, was developed by Dr. Joel Fuhrman. The following index and pyramid shown on the next page is taken directly from his Website, ww.drfuhrman.com/library/article17.aspx. The GERI (Gene Eating Right Index) on my website may be better, in which eggs are 125, olive oil is 36, and milk is 10! Poultry is 36 and coconut oil is 100.

Nutritional science has demonstrated that colorful plant foods contain a huge assortment of protective compounds, most of which still remain unnamed. Only by eating an assortment of nutrient-rich natural foods can we access these protective compounds and prevent the disease and obesity that afflict our current civilization. We need the whole orchestra, not just the woodwinds to make Beethoven's Third Symphony sound wonderful. That is why multi-supplement pills do not work.

Fish contains Omega 3s, which increase insulin sensitivity in muscles and preserves production of the pancreas. The Omega 3s should come from farmed salmon, which has 6,000 mg per six-ounce serving, compared to the wild with 4,500.

Dr. Fuhrman's
ANDI Scoring System: Sample Scores[1]

Kale	1000	Cantaloupe	100	Skim Milk	36
Collards	1000	Kidney Beans	100	Walnuts	34
Bok Choy	824	Sweet Potato	83	Grapes	31
Spinach	739	Black Beans	83	White Potato	31
Broccoli Rabe	715	Sunflower Seeds	78	Banana	30
Chinese/Napa Cabbage	704	Apple	76	Cashews	27
Brussel Sprouts	672	Peach	73	Chicken Breast	27
Swiss Chard	670	Green Peas	70	Eggs	27
Arugula	559	Cherries	68	Peanut Butter	26
Cabbage	481	Flax Seeds	65	Whole Wheat Bread	25
Romaine Lettuce	389	Pineapple	64	Feta Cheese	21
Broccoli	376	Chick Peas	57	Whole Milk	20
Carrot Juice	344	Oatmeal	53	Ground Beef	20
Cauliflower	295	Pumpkin Seeds	52	White Pasta	18
Green Peppers	258	Mango	51	White Bread	18
Artichoke	244	Cucumber	50	Apple Juice	16
Carrots	240	Soybeans	48	Swiss Cheese	15
Asparagus	234	Pistachio Nuts	48	Low Fat Yogurt	14
Strawberries	212	Corn	44	Potato Chips	11
Pomegranate Juice	193	Brown Rice	41	American Cheese	10
Tomato	164	Salmon	39	Vanilla Ice Cream	9
Blueberries	130	Almonds	38	French Fries	7
Iceberg Lettuce	110	Shrimp	38	Olive Oil	2
Orange	109	Avocado	37	Cola	1
Lentils	100	Tofu	37		

HANDY ANDI FOOD PYRAMID

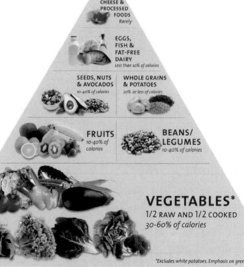

BEEF, SWEETS, CHEESE & PROCESSED FOODS
Rarely

EGGS, FISH & FAT-FREE DAIRY
Less than 10% of calories

SEEDS, NUTS & AVOCADOS
10-40% of calories

WHOLE GRAINS & POTATOES
20% or less of calories

FRUITS
10-40% of calories

BEANS/ LEGUMES
10-40% of calories

VEGETABLES*
1/2 RAW AND 1/2 COOKED
30-60% of calories

Excludes white potatoes. Emphasis on green vegetables

Copyright © 2010 Joel Fuhrman M.D.

*ANDI greater than 200 are on the bottom. These foods are healthier than those that are on the top. Fruits consumed should be mostly berries and cherries.

If these came from Chile, Scandinavia, British Columbia, or Australia, they are without pollution compared to Asian-farmed salmon. Wild fish are not richer in Omega 3 fish oils than farm-raised varieties. Farm-raised fish such as salmon and trout won't grow without Omega 3 fatty acids in their diet, so fish farmers add it to the fish meal. Farmed catfish and tilapia, however, do not need Omega 3 fatty acids, so these farm-raised fish have little or no Omega 3s. In the wild, fish get their Omega 3s from algae, plankton, and other fish that they may eat. The best Omega 3 is DHA from algae like spiralena.

Escolar (ivory tuna) has even more Omega 3s. This essential fat should be consumed as the working DHA and/or EPA rather than ALA, a precursor of the active form that many of us cannot convert to EPA and DHA. Research has shown that Omega 3 fatty acids, particularly DHA, decrease risk of arrhythmias (abnormal heartbeats), which can lead to sudden death. Omega 3 fatty acids also decrease triglyceride levels, raise the super-good cholesterol (HDL-2), slow the growth rate of atherosclerotic plaque, and lowers blood pressure. Fish is also a good source of protein, and unlike fatty meat products, it's not high in saturated fat. Although they have had a bad reputation in the past, tropical oils (palm kernel, palm, and significantly coconut) are saturated fats, but they are metabolized to medium-chain triglycerides, which produce healthy nutritional ketosis. These protect our blood vessels, do not go into our fat cells, and are used by our body to enhance the functioning of our heart and skeletal muscle as well as our neurons.

Some types of fish may contain high levels of mercury, PCBs, dioxins and other environmental contaminants. Levels of these substances are generally highest in older, larger predatory fish. Avoid eating those fish; they have the potential for the highest level of mercury contamination (e.g., shark, swordfish, king mackerel, or tilefish). Eat a variety of fish and shellfish that are lower in mercury (escolar, salmon, canned light tuna, pollock, and catfish). Albacore ("white") tuna has more mercury than canned. Check local advisories about the safety of fish that you might catch yourself from local lakes, rivers, and coastal areas. It is well documented by research that selenium in many of these fish or by ingesting this mineral pulls mercury out of the body (see page 308). Perchlorate, an ingredient in rocket fuel, has infiltrated 80 percent of our inland farm streams and ponds. It is a thyroid receptor inhibiter, causing low thyroid in millions of folks who are being told by doctors that there is nothing wrong with them. This (Type II) hypothyroid does not show up on any of the modern blood studies, but it does on the old-fashioned BMR (Basic Metabolism Rate), which is still done by only a handful of physicians in our modern, highly technical medical society.

In summary, a non-red meat (such as fish) and high-nutrient dense vegetable-based diet offers a healthy protein, high Omega 3s, and lower refined carbohydrates. This program emphasizes a liberal intake of vegetables, some beans, a few tree nuts, but it is low in high glycemic fruits and minimal grains and almost no bad carbs (sugar and starch). Weight loss is sustained in patients who followed this. Favorable changes in the lipid profile and blood pressure are common. In fact in our successful patients who were hypertensive, diabetic, and had bad lipids, we were able to "cure" them of their disease and stop all their medications! This diet has the potential to provide sustainable, and significant, long-term weight loss, and provides substantial lowering of cardiac risk and potential disabilities in patients who are so motivated.

Genetic Reactions to Food

Prior to the development of agriculture approximately twelve thousand years ago, we were hunters and gatherers. According to some experts, grains, dairy products, and refined sugars are the bane of human existence. These were not in the diet of our ancient ancestors, nor were they present in the Garden of Eden. The meats consumed were lean, coming from wild game. Because the animals consumed ate grass, they possessed the healthy CLA, which further allowed humans to convert fat to muscle. Gathered foods were also low in fat and high in fiber. Different blood and body types developed in response to these food sources and lifestyles. The oldest blood type of the human race is type O.

On the Savannah plains of Africa where, according to Dr. Peter J. D'Adamo, humans developed, survival depended on intense physical exercise and animal protein. These ancient people were primarily hunters. Thus, they ate virtually no dairy products and only negligible amounts of grain. Then, through evolution and migration, blood type A developed. These people subsisted on a vegetarian diet since they were foremost gatherers and poor hunters. Blood type B developed later with animal husbandry and milk production. These people had strong digestive systems that could tolerate both animal and vegetable proteins. The most recent in terms of evolution is the rare blood type AB. Because these humans are biologically more complex, they can eat some foods from the A group as well as the B group.

According to Dr. D'Adamo there are six body types: the hunter, the explorer, the teacher, the warrior, the gatherer, and the nomad. He uses anthropomorphic measurements, not just body typing or other systems of metabolic typing. Dimensions of head circumference, finger lengths, height, arm span, sitting height, etc., are included in his relook at the blood types. These are well described in his book, *Eat Right 4 Your Blood Type*, although it is a bit cumbersome to follow.

Though our lifestyle is no longer dominated by how we obtain our food, the correlation between diet, blood type, and body type is still strong. When people eat correctly for their blood type, they not only feel better, but they also have fewer

TABLE 3-I
BLOOD TYPE AND FOOD TO AVOID

TYPE O—MOST COMMON

Meats/Seafood — Goose, barracuda, catfish, caviar, conch, lox, octopus, pickled herring, all pork

Eggs/Dairy — American cheese, blue cheese, brie, buttermilk, camembert, casein, cheddar, colby, cottage cheese, cream cheese, edam, emmenthal, goat milk, gouda, gruyere, ice cream, jarlsberg, kefir, monterey jack, munster, parmesan, provolone, neufchatel, ricotta, skim or 2% milk, string cheese, swiss, whole milk, yogurt (all varieties)

Oils/Fats/Nuts/Seeds — Corn oil, cottonseed oil, peanut, safflower oil, brazil nuts, cashews, lichi, peanuts, peanut butter, pistachios, poppy seeds

Beans — Copper, kidney, navy and tamarind beans; domestic, green and red lentils

Cereals/Bread/Grains/Pasta — Cornflakes, cornmeal, cream of wheat, familia, farina, grape nuts, oat bran, oatmeal, seven-grain, shredded wheat, wheat bran, wheat germ, wheat bagels, corn muffins durum wheat, english muffins, high-protein bread, wheat matzos, multi-grain bread, oat bran muffins, pumpernickel, wheat bran muffins, whole wheat bread, bulgur wheat flour, coucous flour, gluten flour, graham flour, oat flour, soba noodles, semolina and spinach pasta, white and whole wheat flour

Vegetables/Fruits — CA avocado; brussel sprouts, chinese, the red and white cabbage; cauliflower; white and yellow corn; eggplant; domestic and shitake mushrooms, mustard greens; black, greek and spanish olives; red and white potatoes; alfalfa sprouts; blackberries; coconuts; cantaloupe and honeydew melon; oranges; plantains; rhubarb; tangerines; apple juice and cider; cabbage juice; orange juice

Spices/Condiments — Capers; cinnamon; cornstarch; corn syrup; nutmeg; black and white pepper; apple cider, balsamic, red wine and white vinegar; ketchup; dill, kosher, sweet and sour pickles; relish

Beverages — Coffee, distilled liquor, sodas, black tea.

TYPE A — COMMON

Meats/Fish/Seafood — Beef, buffalo, duck, goose, heart, lamb, liver, mutton, partridge, pheasant, all pork, rabbit, veal, venison, quail, anchovy, barracuda, beluga, bluefish, bluegill, bass, catfish, caviar, clam, conch, crab, crayfish, eel, flounder, frog, gray sole, haddock, haka, halibut, herring (fresh or pickled), lobster, lox, mussels, octopus, oysters, scallop, shad, shrimp, sole, squid, striped bass, tilefish, turtle

Eggs/Dairy — American cheese, blue cheese, brie, butter, buttermilk, camembert, casein, cheddar, colby, cottage, cream cheese, edam, emmenthal, gouda, gruyere, ice cream, jarlsberg, monterey jack, munster, neufchatel, parmesan, provolone, sherbet, skim or 2% milk, sour cream (non-fat), swiss, whole milk

Oils/Fats/Nuts/Seeds — Corn, cottonseed oil, peanut, safflower oil; brazil nuts, cashews, pistachios

Beans — Copper, garbanzo, kidney, lima, navy, red, tamarind

Cereals/Bread/Grains/Pasta — Cream of wheat, familia, farina, granola, grape nuts, wheat germs, seven grain, shredded wheat, wheat bran, durum wheat, english muffins, high-protein bread, wheat matzos, pumpernickel, wheat bran muffins, whole wheat bread, whole wheat and white flour, semolina pasta, spinach pasta

Vegetables/Fruits — Chinese, red and white cabbage; eggplant; domestic and shitake mushrooms; black, greek and spanish olives; green, red, yellow and jalapeno peppers; sweet, red and white potatoes; yams; tomatoes; bananas; coconuts; mangoes; cantaloupe and honeydew melon; oranges; papayas; plantains; rhubarb; tangerines; orange juice; papaya juice; tomato juice

Spices/Condiments — Capers; gelatin; black, cayenne, peppercorn, red and white pepper; apple cider, balsamic, red or white vinegar; wintergreen; ketchup; mayonnaise; tabasco, worcestershire sauce

Beverages — Beer, liquor, sodas, black tea (regular or decaffeinated)

TYPE B — RARE

Meats/Fish/Seafood — Chicken, cornish hens, duck, goose, heart, partridge, all pork, quail, anchovy, barracuda, beluga, bluegill, bass, clam, conch, crab, crayfish, eel, farm-raised salmon, frog, lobster, lox, mussels, octopus, oysters, sea bass, shrimp, snail, striped bass, turtle, yellowtail

Eggs/Dairy — American cheese, blue cheese, ice cream, string cheese

Oils/Fats/Nuts/Seeds — Canola oil, corn oil, cottonseed oil, peanut oil, safflower oil, sesame oil, sunflower oil, cashews, filberts, pignola, pistachio, peanuts, peanut butter, poppy seeds, pumpkin seeds, sesame butter and seeds, tahini, sunflower seeds

Beans — Aduke; azuki; black; garbanzo; pinto; domestic, green and red lentils; black-eyed peas

Cereals/Bread/Grains/Pasta — Amaranth, barley, buckwheat, cornflakes, cornmeal, cream of wheat, kamut, kasha, rye, seven-grain, shredded wheat, wheat bran, wheat germ, wheat bagels, corn muffins, durum wheat, multi-grain bread, 100% rye bread, rye crisp, rye vita, wheat bran muffins, whole wheat floor, buckwheat, coucous, artichoke pasta, wild rice, gluten flour, soba noodles

Vegetables/Fruits — Domestic and jerusalem artichoke, CA avocado, white and yellow corn; black, greek and spanish olives; pumpkin, radishes, sprouts, tempeh, tofu, tomato, coconuts, persimmons, pomegranate, prickly pear, rhubarb, starfruit, mung sprouts

Spices/Condiments — Allspice, almond extract, barley malt, cinnamon, cornstarch, corn syrup, ketchup, plain gelatin, black ground and white pepper, tapioca, all spices; capers

Beverages — Distilled liquor, sodas

TYPE AB — — — VERY RARE

Meats/Fish/Seafood — Beef, buffalo, chicken, cornish hens, duck, goose, heart, partridge, all pork, venison, quail, anchovy, barracuda, beluga, bluegill, bass, clam, conch, crab, crayfish, eel, farm-raised salmon, flounder, frog, gray sole, haddock, halibut, pickled herring, lobster, lox, octopus, oysters, sea bass, shrimp, striped bass, turtle, yellowtail

Eggs/Dairy — American cheese, blue cheese, brie, butter, buttermilk, camembert, ice cream, parmesan, provolone, sherbet, whole milk

Oils/Fats/Nuts/Seeds — Corn oil, cotton-seed oil, peanut oil, safflower oil, sesame oil, sunflower oil, filberts, poppy seeds, pumpkin seeds, sesame seeds, tahini, sunflower seeds

Beans — Aduke; azuki; black; fava, garbanzo; kidney; lima; black-eyed peas

Cereals/Bread/Grains/Pasta — Buckwheat, corn, kamut, kasha, corn muffins, artichoke pasta, soba noodles

Vegetables/Fruits — Domestic and jerusalem artichoke, CA avocado, white and yellow corn; abalone and shitake mushrooms, black olives, green, red and yellow peppers, jalapeno peppers, radishes, radish sprouts, mung sprouts, bananas, coconuts, guava, mangoes, oranges, persimmons, pomegranate, prickly pear, rhubarb, starfruit

Spices/Condiments — Allspice, almond extract, anise, barley malt, capers, cornstarch, corn syrup; black, cayenne pepper (black, cayenne, red flakes, peppercorn), tapioca, vinegar (balsamic, red or white), ketchup, pickles (kosher, sweet, sour), relish, worcestershire sauce

Beverages — Distilled liquor, sodas, black tea

(If appropriate, xerox and cut out your blood type to carry in your wallet.)

degenerative diseases (e.g., cardiovascular disease, obesity, arthritis), allergies, and cancer. It should be noted that an A, B, or O blood type has nothing to do with whether one is rh positive (e.g., O+) or negative (e.g., A-). Although I am not as bullish on the blood and body types as I have been in the past, there is some validity in them. Look at the chart on the previous page and "if the shoe fits, wear it."

Food Reactions

A true food allergy originates in the white blood cells (lymphocytes) and internal lining cells. If one eats a food against which the body has developed a specific antibody group, an explosive reaction takes place. This results in acute inflammation of the skin or nerves, or more serious, a sudden reduction of the airways, or anaphylactic shock (cardiovascular pulmonary collapse), which is occasionally lethal. Shellfish, certain nuts, and strawberries are the most common offenders of this sort and must be completely avoided by people allergic to them.

Food intolerances are a type of allergy and are also the result of bodily incompatibility, but they usually do not call as much attention to themselves. Lactose, fructose, and wheat/gluten intolerances are now well-accepted medical diagnoses. Other hidden food intolerances are not as well accepted, but are nevertheless important in a holistic physician's thinking. They do not cause discernible immediate reactions, but over time subtle symptoms gradually build up. Obesity and degenerative diseases can be attributed to this phenomenon, as are acne, stuffy nose, irritable bowel, recurrent respiratory infection, migraines, muscle aches, ADHD, and fatigue.

Methodically eliminating individual foods is the do-it-yourself method of identifying specific food intolerances. This, however, is time-consuming and can be frustrating to someone who has identified the problem but not its source. Fortunately there is an easier way: skin, hydrogen breath test, and blood tests can detect the offending food. The MIR and the ALCAT (Antigen Leukocyte Cellular Antibody Test), found on the web at www.alcat.com. Sage Lab (www.sagelab.com), not only tests specific foods, but breaks down products of these foods, termed peptides. These are the subgroups that cross the intestines and cause mischief. The Immunocap by Phadia (www.phadia.us) tests for immunoglobulin-E (IgE)-mediated food allergies for various foods and inhaled substances.

Large Waist, Short Life

Apart from glamorized body images in advertising and magazines, there are medical standards of appropriate weight. Thus, when patients ask me, "What should I weigh?" we discuss their ideal weight; the body mass index (BMI), which relates size to weight in a numerical value; percent body fat; and waist to hip ratio (WHR). The ideal BMI is less than 25; the ideal percent body fat is 15 percent for males and 22 percent for females. The truism "large waist, short life" applies if the WHR is greater than 1.0 for a man, and .85 for a woman. Though these may sound like aesthetic measurements, they are not. Excessive abdominal girth, for instance, is associated with abnormalities that cause both morbidity (illness) and mortality (death). The metabolic syndrome is characterized by ear creases, a tendency toward high sugar triglycerides, high blood pressure, low HDL cholesterol, and a large gut. Three or four of these factors are all that some doctors need to make this diagnosis. The intra-abdominal fat cells are not just a storage unit to hold fat, but are actively secreting cytochymes, a damaging chemical that raises CRP (C-reactive protein), the molecule said to destroy blood vessels and cause cancer. Alternatively, we can assess our weight ourselves by standing naked in front of a long mirror. A female at her ideal weight will have little cellulite and no fat rolls, and a male should see his ribs without having love handles below them.

According to recent literature, 33 percent of adults do not pass this test. In some populations, such as Hispanics and Native Americans where I live in Oklahoma, as many as 60 percent are overweight and are developing the metabolic syndrome or its evil sibling, diabetes. The agricultural and industrial revolutions do have a detrimental effect by giving society more food and less physical work than we need.

Eating too much is only part of the problem. Being overweight or obese has both genetic and environmental causes. Paradoxically, when one is over the age of seventy having excess weight may not be so bad. In an article in the *Archives of Internal Medicine*, patients hospitalized with a BMI of greater than 25 had a better outcome than those with less.[2] But if their excess weight were more muscle, their outcomes would be even better.

The mind-set of our society and, unfortunately of many physicians, is, "If fat does not pass my lips, it will not end up on my hips." While it is true that fat is a high calorie food, it is high glycemic carbohydrates that make us fat! Research shows that the prevalence for being overweight rose from 25.4 percent in 1986 to 33.3 percent in 1996—a 31 percent increase! During the same period the average fat intake adjusted for total calories dropped 5 percent. Therefore, reduced fat intake and the frequent consumption of "low calorie" food products is actually associated with an increase of obesity. The *Atkins Low Carb Diet* has now been time tested and has passed peer review in the medical journals to become one of the better ways to prevent fat. Some carbs are okay, but not all carbs are created equal. A glycemic index helps to distinguish the good from the bad and, as mentioned earlier, if a carb is greater than 50, it is *crap* (short for a *crapohydrate*). This does not imply that eating fat indiscriminately is harmless. Fat has nine calories per gram while protein and carbohydrates have only four. Ninety percent of our excess carbohydrates go directly into unsightly storage, rather than being burned for fuel—unless we exercise within one hour of eating.

Part of the problem is that we do not burn enough calories, even with regular exercise. Because of modern transportation and other labor-saving inventions of the last three centuries, our daily lives require less muscle use than in the past. Thus, to stay healthy some of us do "artificial work," deliberate exercise, to make up for our lack of useful physical activity. Aerobic exercise, the sustained use of muscles for twenty to thirty minutes, is good. But anaerobic or resistance exercise like lifting weights and working with a Nautilus-like machine is better.

Despite our genetic programming or the work-saving machines we use on a daily basis, we do not *have* to be overweight or obese. Proper eating practices can counteract these influences, because *how much* we eat is often determined by *how* we eat. We need to practice eating more slowly, tasting and appreciating our food. If you are alone, eat without distractions such as television. Concentrate on the texture, the taste, the temperature, and the nutritional value of the food. And, of course, eat slowly. Chew each bite five to ten times, not just to masticate for ingestion, but to allow the micronutrients in the food to be better absorbed by your digestive processes. When you do this, your intestines, and the intrinsic intestinal hormones there, will tell your brain when you are no longer hungry. Also, eating more slowly allows time to stimulate the hormones such as incretin, a chemical that allows the proper balance of insulin and glucagon from our pancreas. If we eat more slowly, we will also enjoy our food more. Anticipating something pleasant after the meal should lure us away from the table instead of lingering to eat as long as the food exists. It takes approximately twenty minutes for the food in our stomachs to give the message to our brains that we are satiated and do not need to eat more.

Momentum in the Omentum—Inflamation

The omentum is an apron-like, lacy tissue that drops down from the stomach. It is both a fat storehouse and an endocrine organ. It determines our weight and our health from inside the abdominal cavity. The subcutaneous, superficial yellow fat often found in the buttocks, thighs, and abdomen is different in its makeup; it is less active and serves as insulation until our omental fat stores are diminished.

The white fat from the omentum is much more aggressive. The brown fat found around some of our organs and the mid to upper chest regulates thermogenesis, an elusive mechanism that is the key to our weight, and on which much research is being done. The omentum releases the hormone leptin (Greek for "thin"), which tells the brain how full we feel.

Overweight people have less of the hormone leptin; therefore they don't feel full as quickly or as often. This leads them to eat more than they should, causing them to become more overweight. The omentum also secretes interleukin 6, which goes directly to the liver and stimulates C-reactive protein (CRP) production. This specifically damages our arteries. The body's endo-cannabinoid system (ECS) controls food intake and energy expenditure, and it has its receptor in the omentum. Triglyceride is found in both the omentum and the blood and figures into both good cholesterol levels and insulin resistance.

In general, the bigger the omentum, the higher the blood triglycerides. The lower the healthy HDL cholesterol, the more the insulin resistance, and the greater the likelihood of cardiometabolic syndrome and diabetes.

Once the omentum is filled with fat, it leaks some to the liver, which gradually destroys it. An epidemic of NASH (NonAlcoholic SteatoHepatosis) is occurring in the United States. This is a condition in which initially there is a slight increase of liver enzymes (AST, ALT), later fibrosis, and even cirrhosis of the liver. The liver becomes sluggish and doesn't detoxify the internal and external chemicals as it should. This plays a role in various illnesses, including cancer.

Intra-abdominal adiposity, a reflection of omental size, can be calculated with an abdominal CT scan. However, it is easier to measure the waist, which for a woman, should be less than 32.5 inches, or 35 inches for a man. The larger the waist size, the more you are at risk for all causes of mortality, including stroke, heart attack, and cancer. Your girth (waist size) is more important than your weight. The best way to determine intra-abdominal adiposity is the WHR (waist-hip ratio) in which less than 1 for a man or .85 for a woman is healthy.

Obesity is a more complex condition than being over-weight; it is, in fact, a disease. It is not caused merely by a lack of willpower, slovenliness, or gluttony, but by a neuro-hormonal imbalance, genetically endowed and environmentally nurtured. Obesity is actually the most common form of malnutrition in our modern society, resulting from an improper complement of macro- and micronutrients. According to the law of natural thermodynamics, if we ingest more calories than we can burn off, we store the excess in the form of fat. Excess fat is mentally and physically destructive. It decreases neural transmission and may even lower IQ. Obese people have a much higher incidence of degenerative diseases such as cardio-vascular and metabolic disease (diabetes, gout, etc.), arthritis, Alzheimer's and cancer, especially of the colon, breast, and uterus.

Injectable human chorio-gonadotropin (HcG) and other lipotropics such as methionine choline and inositol have been proven helpful in my practice. These mobilize the fat out of the liver to be "burned," allowing the liver to function better. In morbidly obese refractory cases in which the individual has yo-yoed many times, I frequently recommend surgical bypass procedures. It is an effective way to lose weight, but it is costly and does have a risk of complications such as blood clots to the lungs and, occasionally, death. Gastric banding has been done with laparotomy for the last twenty years, without major surgery through an incision in the abdomen. This is now possible in some institutions as an outpatient. An inflatable water girdle is inserted through a small keyhole in the abdomen. Its volume of water can then be adjusted as needed with a needle placed through the skin to enlarge or decrease the stomach volume.

For now, there is no magic solution for weight loss, but everyone can lose weight by following these guidelines: Go easy on crapohydrates; eat slowly, and only until you are satisfied rather than stuffed; and do not skip meals. For weight control, six small meals, with the largest at breakfast, are better than one large meal in the evening. Most importantly, we must exercise. The law of natural thermodynamics is simple and clear: If we burn more calories than we consume, we will lose weight.

FOOD FROM THE SEA

Nutrition under the sea is not about eating fish, but that which the fish eats—the vegetables (seaweed, algae, and kelp). Sea vegetables are commonly eaten by humans in Asian cultures. Edible seaweeds have steadily increased in popularity since the 1980s, no doubt in a large part due to the rise in popularity of sushi. The sushi, or maki-sushi, consists of rice and raw fish wrapped in delicious and healthful sea vegetables, such as dulse and wakame.

Omega 3s from fish is a fantastically healthful product, but better is DHA from algae. It not only helps people to lose weight but lowers blood pressure and contributes to heart health and mental health. The long-lived Okinawans, who have very little if any chronic disease, consume the most seaweed per capita of any place in the world. Seaweed is chockful of vitamins, minerals, protein, as well as DHA fiber. The dietary fiber derived from sea vegetables has an anti-cancer, a fat-diminishing, and a mild anticoagulant effect, as well as being a super-antioxidant. The best, is spirulina, a freshwater green algae that assists in bowel health, heart health, and the reduction of heavy metal toxicity. Spirulina contains many carotenoids and antioxidants plus the ideal protein (far better than milk) along with other super-micronutrients.

DHA from algae is a supplement from the Martek Corporation. Edible seaweed is available in most Asian grocery and health food stores. It usually comes in a dry form and is made "fresh" again by simply soaking in water. There are hundreds of ways to use these products, such as in salads, in soups, and as a vegetable dish. It can also be added to gravies, casseroles, or cereal. It can be pickled and used as a condiment, or as a spice in vegetable dishes. It is the main component of a popular Japanese soup stock called Dashi. Arame is known for its mild, almost sweet flavor, and it can be added to soups or salads or steamed or boiled and eaten plain. Wakame is a green, slightly "fishy" seaweed. According to investigators at Notre Dame Seishin University in Japan, this sea vegetable increases magnesium, which is low in most of us. "Under the Sea Food" is the up and coming future food and should be a part of everyone's diet. Why wait for it to become "popular"? Add it to your diet today!

THE MESSAGE ON THE BOTTLE

The container that holds and is used while heating liquids or solid food, as well as water, may be more important than its contents. In the last three decades, there has been a 500 percent increase of plastics used in our immediate environment. The three worst offenders are phthalates, biphenol A, and Styrofoam. These are hormone (estrogen, thyroid) disrupters, binding to their receptors. Also the Styrofoam hydrocarbons in cups or other bottles can cause cancer.

Phthalates, or phthalate esters, are ubiquitous and mainly

Plastic Resin Recycling Codes

Polyethylene Terephthalate (PET)	High Density Polyethylene (HDPE)	Polyvinyl Chloride (PVC)
♲ 1	♲ 2	♲ 3
PETE	HDPE	V

Low Density Polyethylene (LDPE)	Polypropylene (PP)	Polystyrene (PS)
♲ 4	♲ 5	♲ 6
LDPE	PP	PS

Several Other Plastics Some Unknown (BAD)

♲ 7

OTHER

used as plasticizers (substances added to plastics to increase their flexibility, transparency, durability, and longevity). They are primarily used to soften polyvinyl chloride. Phthalates are being phased out of many products in the United States and the European Union due to various health concerns. However, they are still used in a large variety of non-container products, from enteric coatings of pharmaceutical pills and nutritional supplements for viscosity control, gelling agents, film formers, stabilizers, dispersants, lubricants, binders, emulsifiers, and suspending agents. End products include adhesives and glues, agricultural additives, building materials, personal care products, medical devices, detergents and surfactants, packaging, children's toys, modeling clay, waxes, paints, printing inks and coatings, pharmaceuticals, food products, and textiles.

Phthalates are also frequently used in soft plastic fishing lures, caulk, paint pigments, and sex toys made of so-called jelly rubber. Phthalates are used in a variety of household applications used in shower curtains, vinyl upholstery, adhesives, floor tiles, food containers and wrappers, and cleaning materials. Personal care items containing phthalates include perfume, eye shadow, moisturizer, nail polish, liquid soap, and hair spray. They are also found in modern electronics and medical applications such as catheters and blood transfusion devices. The most widely used phthalates are the di-2-ethylhexyl phthalate (DEHP), the diisodecyl phthalate (DIDP), and the diisononyl phthalate (DINP). DEHP is the dominant plasticizer used in PVC due to its low cost. Butyl benzyl phthalate (BBP) is used in the manufacture of foamed PVC, which is mostly employed as a flooring material. Phthalates with small "R and R" groups (attached organic molecules) are used as solvents in perfumes and pesticides.

Phthalates are easily released into the environment because there is no covalent bond between the chemicals and the plastic in which they are mixed. As plastics age and break down, the release of phthalates accelerates. Phthalates in the environment are subject to biodegradation, photodegradation, and anaerobic degradation and therefore they do not generally persist long in an outdoor environment. Indoor air concentrations, however, are a different story. Their concentrations vary with the age and nature of the sources. Because of their volatility, DEP and DMP are present in higher concentrations in air in comparison with the heavier and less volatile DEHP. Higher air temperatures result in higher concentrations of phthalates. PVC flooring leads to higher density of BBP and DEHP, which are more prevalent in dust.

As you can imagine, people are commonly exposed to phthalates, and most Americans tested by the Centers for Disease Control and Prevention have metabolites of multiple phthalates in their urine. Because phthalate plasticizers are not chemically bound to PVC, they can easily leach and evaporate into food or the atmosphere. Phthalate exposure can occur through direct use or indirectly through leaching and general environmental contamination. In the Midwest, many fish in streams are banned from human consumption because of the adulteration of the water by public and private landfills. Diet is believed to be the main source of DEHP and other phthalates in the general population. Fatty foods such as milk, butter, and meats are a major source of toxicity, since they more rapidly absorb these lypophillic (fat-loving) chemicals. Low molecular weight phthalates such as DEP, DBP, and BBzP are absorbed through the skin. Inhalational exposure is also more significant with the more volatile phthalates.

The actual risks of BPA are still a matter of public debate, but over the past decade, a growing body of scientific studies has linked the chemical to breast and prostrate cancer, infertility, obesity, as well as neurological and behavioral changes, including autism and hyperactivity. Bisphenol A is also an endocrine disruptor; it can mimic the body's own hormones, which may lead to negative health effects if the dosage is high. There are theories that it may contribute to body fat. A September 2008 study in the *Journal of the American Medical Association* found that higher levels of urinary BPA is associated with cardiovascular disease, diabetes, and liver-enzyme abnormalities. "Tin" cans are coated with BPA on the inside. The acid and fat in foods enhance absorption of these and are accelerated if one heats the food in the can.

Styrene is made from benzene, which has been clearly shown to be carcinogenic. The migration of styrene from a polystyrene cup into the beverage it contains has been observed to be as high as 0.025 percent for a single use. That may seem like a rather low number until you work it out. If you drink beverages from polystyrene cups four times a day for three years you may have consumed about one foam cup of styrene along with your beverages. Styrene migration has been shown to be partially dependent on the heat and fat content of the food in the polystyrene cups/containers—the higher the fat content and the temperature, the higher the migration into the food. Entrees, soups, or beverages that are higher in fat (like a bowl of three-cheese chili or tall cupful of Triple-Cream Frappa-Mocha Java Delight) will suck much more of the styrene out of the polystyrene container than water. Some compounds found in beverages, like alcohol or the acids in "tea with lemon," may also raise the styrene migration rate.

Plastic Code Identification: Containers with a 3, 6, or 7 on the bottom are the most dangerous of all. They contain a dangerous and volatile chemical called BPA, and should be avoided at all costs. Containers with a 4 or 5 on the bottom are generally considered safe, but you should probably use them sparingly.

Containers with a 1 or 2 on the bottom are the safest. These include clear water containers, as well as most cloudy containers you normally find containing water or milk. These containers, made from PET, PETE, and HDPE, are safe for storing cold food and drink, but you should never use them in the microwave.

The #7 recycling label is a catch-all indicator for plastics made with a resin other than those in the #1 to #6 designations or is made of more than one resin. The #7 category not only includes polycarbonate but also includes compostable plastics made of organic material and other types of plastic that do not necessarily contain BPA (Bisphenol-A). For example, the new Everyday Line manufactured with Eastman's Tritan copolyester is a #7, but does not include BPA.

Of all the seven grades of commercial plastics available to manufacturers on today's market, unlucky #7 has the worst track record for leaching BPA into liquids or foods likely to be consumed by humans or animals. The reason is because, unlike the other six composites, containers bearing the #7 are made of a composite of leftover scraps that have been "repurposed" and most likely purchased at a discount. The new Nalgene water

PLASTIC IDENTIFICATION CODE	TYPE OF PLASTIC POLYMER	COMMON PACKAGING APPLICATIONS	OK WITH FOOD?
01 PET	POLYETHYLENE TEREPHTHALATE (PET, PETE)	PETE goes into soft drink, juice, water, detergent, and cleaner bottles. Also used for cooking and peanut butter Jars.	YES
02 PE-HD	HIGH DENSITY POLYETHYLENE (HDPE)	High Density Polyethylene HDPE goes into milk and water jugs, bleach bottles, detergent bottles, shampoo bottles, and grocery sacks, motor oil bottles, house hold cleaners.	YES
03 PVC	POLYVINYL CHLORIDE (PVC)	PVC goes into window cleaner, cooking oils, and detergent bottles. Also used for peanut butter jars and water jugs.	BETTER TO AVOID
04 PE-LD	LOW DENSITY POLYETHYLENE (LDPE)	LDPE goes into plastic bags and grocery sacks, dry cleaning bags, flexible film packaging, and some bottles	YES
05 PP	POLYETHYLENE (PP)	PP goes into caps, disks, syrup bottles, yogurt tubs, straws, and film packaging	YES
06 PS	POLYSTYRENE (PS)	PS goes into meat trays, egg cartons, plates, cutlery, carry-out containers, and clear trays.	BETTER TO AVOID
07 O	OTHER: INCULDES POLYCARBONATE	Includes resins not mentioned above or combinations of plastics.	BETTER TO AVOID

bottle is made of a "copolyester" plastic, manufactured by the Eastman Company, with the trade name Tritan. So are new bottles by Kor and Campelbak. All trumpet the fact that their bottles are BPA-free, with the implication that *BPA-free* is the equivalent of *safe*. But there is no way of knowing because the ingredients that make up Tritan have been kept secret. They could include another dangerous chemical. All that is known about the Tritan bottles is that, like polycarbonate, they fall into the #7 category of "other" plastics in the identification system.

When purchasing cling-wrapped food from the supermarket or deli, I recommend that you slice off a thin layer where the food came into contact with the plastic and store the rest in a glass or ceramic container or wrap it in non-PVC cling wrap. Avoid storing fatty foods, such as meat and cheese, in plastic containers or plastic wrap. Hand-wash reusable containers gently with a nonabrasive soap; dishwashers and harsh detergents can scratch plastic, making hospitable homes for bacteria and creating more surface area for toxin dissemination.

"Microwave-safe" or "microwavable" labels on a plastic container only means that it should not melt, crack, or fall apart when used in the microwave. The label is no guarantee that containers don't leach chemicals into foods when heated. Use glass or ceramic containers instead. Some scientists feel that microwaves change the healthy vibrational frequency of the food to an unnatural one which is less compatible with our digestive and metabolic systems.

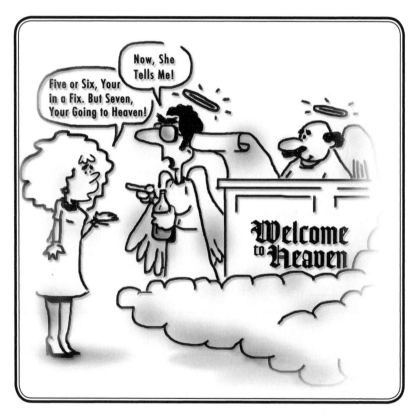

4

MACRONUTRIENTS

FATS OF LIFE

The right fats in the right amounts are not only good for us, but essential. According to a Harvard health study recently published in the *Journal of the American Medical Association*, there was an inverse association between dietary fats and development of strokes in men. Fat is an essential element in our diet. It causes the secretion of CCK (cholecyctokin), which stops the hunger sensation. Our bodies cannot make certain fats—referred to as "essential fatty acids" which we have to get them from our food. Eicosanoids, or prostaglandins (a major chemical transmitter), HDL, cholesterol, hormones, brain tissue, and membranes lining every cell of the body are composed of fat molecules. Furthermore, we need fat for insulation, energy stores and, most importantly, for life itself. A drastic decrease of what is known as "brown fat" is directly correlated with death. Fats also make food more palatable. However, all fats are not created equal. They range from the excellent to the good, the bad, and the very bad.

THE GOOD, THE BAD, THE UGLY, THE HORRIBLE, AND THE EVIL

Excellent:

Omega 3s (DHA): Found in fish and seaweed.

Good:

1. **Gamalinolenic Acid** (GLA): Found in oatmeal, mother's

milk, evening primrose oil, and borage oil. (Omega 3s + GLA increase the good ecosinoids.)

2. **B Sitostanol**: Found in plant sources; lowers cholesterol and possibly reduces prostate size and risk of cancer

3. **Tropical Fats**: Coconut oil and palm kernal oil improve brain and muscle function and are not fattening.

Neutral:

1. **Monounsaturated fats**: These are not nearly as beneficial as the "excellent" fats. The richest source of monounsaturated fats is macadamia nuts, but it is also found in pistachios, walnuts, cashews, and almonds, as well as avocados. Olives, flax, rapeseed (canola), and their oils, and to a lesser extent, peanuts and their oil, have some monounsaturated fats.

2. **Non-absorbable fats**: These fats, such as Simplese and Olestra, do not help the system, but they do not hurt it, either. They do, however, leach out fat soluble micronutrients.

3. **Cholesterol**: It is not the cholesterol we eat, but the cholesterol our body produces in response to what we eat that is bad. If it is oxidized, such as the yolk of a scrambled egg, it can promote atherosclerosis.

Bad:

1. **Polyunsaturates**: These fats, such as corn oil or safflower seed oil, are referred to by nutritionists as Omega 6 fatty acids.

2. **Saturated fats**: These are found in meats.

Very Bad:

1. **Overheated oils**: These promote free radicals.

2. **Hydrogenated vegetable oil**: This contains the trans-polyunsaturates that directly promote atherosclerosis.

3. **Homogenized milk fat**: This contains microglobules of fat that are foreign to our bodies.

Evil:

1. **Burnt and saturated fats:** These contain ALE (Advanced Lipid End Products), as in the grilled fat of "delicious" steak.

Table 3-IV
FATTY ACIDS

Omega 3 series — Alpha Linolenic Acid, Eicosstrienoic Acid, Eicosapentaenoic Acid, Docosahexaenoic Acid

Omega 6 series — Linoleic Acid, Gamma Linolenic Acid, Eicosadienoic Acid, Dihomo-Gammalinoleic Acid, Arachidonic Acid, Docosatetranoic Acid

Omega 9 series — Trans Elaidic Acid, Dis Oleic Acid Eicosenoic Acid, Euricic Acid, Nervonic Acid

Saturated — Palmitic Acid, Stearic Acid

FAT FACTS

The trans-fatty acid data is now well established. A landmark study, published in the *New England Journal of Medicine*, demonstrated that the consumption of products low in trans-fatty acids, (the opposite of cis-fatty acids), will reduce cholesterol and triglycerides. Trans-fatty acids include partially and fully hydrogenated fats, literally from another world. They are man-made, with catalysts such as nickel in the presence of hydrogen, and our bodies do not know how to metabolize them. Although they have been approved by the FDA as a "safe food additive," they truly are a transgression. They are now being legislated out of our diets, starting with New York City and now being adopted by other jurisdictions.

Also bad are oil fats, and cholesterol heated to excess. This decomposes them and turns them into free radical pro-oxidants. They are directly absorbed by the intestines and immediately enter the bloodstream, affecting the lining of blood vessels and causing a buildup of plaque by oxidizing the LDL cholesterol.

On the other hand, numerous studies have shown that consuming seaweed and fish, which contains Omega 3s, decreases the incident of heart attacks and strokes. The Eskimo Paradox, studied almost fifty years ago, is a revealing testimony of this. Despite the fact that their diet was overly rich in fatty foods, including *animal* fat (blubber and seal meat) and fatty fish such as salmon, the Eskimos had healthy cardiovascular systems. The enigma was resolved when we began to understand the strong impact of marine oils on health.

Marine oils are among the seventeen essential fatty acids that must be consumed since our bodies can make only minimal amounts (see Table 3-3). Omega 3s protect the lining of the blood vessels from building up plaque, reduce triglycerides, decrease clotting, and improve the flow of blood. They also play important roles outside the cardiovascular system: in brain functioning, neurotransmitters, the retina, and improving the interaction of almost every cell in our bodies. A double-blind study published in the *Archives of General Psychiatry* showed ninety-six grams of fish oil greatly improved bipolar (manic-depressive) disorder. The cellular membrane (the substance that keeps the inside of the cell inside and functioning) is composed mostly of these essential fatty acids. Also, the lining of our joints and our skin are kept healthy by the Omega 3s. As noted above, DHA is the best.

Nothing Fishy About That

Fish oils and algae are weight-reducing and have other healthy benefits such as the prevention of fatal and non-fatal arrhythmias, stroke, heart attacks, Alzheimer's, and depression. As a fringe benefit, it keeps the skin younger than its years. According to an article published in *Lancet*, fish oil (Omega 3 fatty acids) stabilized atherosclerotic plaques. Plaque is an accumulation of cells or cell debris that contain lipids (cholesterol and fatty acids), calcium, and a variable amount of fibrous connective tissue. Plaque is an unhealthy condition. Cardiovascular disease is related to plaque in blood vessels.

In half of all first heart attacks, plaque doesn't block or occlude blood vessels. Plaque, which is inherently unstable, can release fragments that lodge in smaller blood vessels, causing hemorrhaging plus significant and sudden narrowing of the vessel. A clot that forms on top of a leaky plaque may occlude the vessel. Even though it may block 60 percent of the vessel, a stable plaque is not dangerous. By either direct pathologic examination or with the assistance of ultrasound, doctors can classify a plaque as being stable (calcified) or unstable (soft).

In a well-designed double-blind clinical trial, a variety of fats were given to 162 patients scheduled to undergo a carotid endarterectomy for advanced arteriosclerosis. One-third of the patients were given Omega 3 fatty acids, another third were given Omega 6 (vegetable oil), and another third were given capsules that contained the mixtures of oils comparable to a typical Western diet. During surgery, sections were taken from the artery and classified by a cardiopathologist as either unstable or stable. The ones who consumed the westernized diet oils or the Omega 6s had greater than 50 percent more unstable plaques compared to those who were given the Omega 3 fatty acids.

The bottom line is to increase dietary Omega fats by consuming oil-bearing fish such as salmon or escolar, and as supplements of DHA. Although a capsule may have on the label 1000 or even 1200 mg, the active DHA and EPA may be together only 300 mg and the DHA 125! So one needs to consume 10 to 20 of them to get a decent dose. Although Krill

Oil has been touted to be as good if not better than fish oil. I have found it not nearly as good. Omega 3s are also available in liquids. They are now not only very concentrated but even palatable. Also as noted above, sea weed/algae are very high in these healthy oils. After all, that is where the fish get theirs. The best Omega 3 is DHA (DexaHexinoic Acid), which is three times more beneficial than EPA (Eicospentoic Acoid). There is also ALA (Alpha Linolenic Acid) in flax and primrose. Although classified as an Omega 3, it is a *pre* Omega 3, and our metabolism converts it into the active DHA if it can. Unfortunately, this is only true if we are young (under twenty-five) and healthy.

Eating a high fat or protein diet is certainly better than eating crapohydrates. But watch the type of fat you eat. It is said that eating one pound of hydrogenated fat will allow you to gain one pound since the body needs to dilute this bad fat by holding onto other fat. One pound of saturated fat will give a weight gain of one-quarter pound, but eating one pound of Omega 3s will cause one-quarter pound of weight loss in that it recycles into your cellular membranes and discharges the previous fat residing there for excretion into the bile.Now one can track their Omega 3s by a special red cell fatty acid test offered by Spectracel. This reflects three months of not only consumption but absorption and utilization of this healthy nutrient.

CLA Will Make Your Day

CLA, conjugated linoleic acid, is a natural polyunsaturated fatty acid found in many foods, including milk, cheese, and meats. The meat richest in CLA is beef, but it is also found in lamb and veal and, to a lesser degree, in pork, chicken, and turkey. CLA is made in the bellies of ruminants such as cows from grass fermented with the help of certain bacteria (bacteritites). In a study of CLA content under various feeding regimens, cows allowed to graze freely on the range had 500 percent more CLA in their milk fat than cows fed typical dairy farm diets supplemented with corn silage or grain. CLA concentration is further increased when meats are cooked.

Evidence compiled over the last two decades has led to the recognition that CLA possesses unique and potent antioxidant, anticarcinogenic (antiatherosclerotic), and anticatabolic (helping to prevent metabolic destructiveness) effects. It is taken up by the body's phospholipids, a class of fats that serves as the principal structural components of cell membranes. CLA is now thought to represent a previously unidentified defense mechanism against membrane attack by oxygen radicals. It enhances body composition by increasing muscle while reducing fat. Moreover, in animal studies, CLA has been shown to increase bone mass and exert a positive effect on diabetes by increasing insulin sensitivity.

CLA is produced synthetically by heating linoleic acid (an essential nutrient found widely in plant oils and animal fats) in the presence of a base. CLA increases HD=2, cholesterol and decreases LDL and triglycerides. CLA modulates leukotrienes, which suppress the immunoglobin associated with allergies.

Although one can obtain neutral CLA from seared meats (which also contain ALE), I recommend concentrated sources. CLA comes in 1000 mg doses taken daily and costs about a dollar a capsule. This is very safe, and doses of 4000 mg a day are used to increase muscle, decrease fat, and improve the immune function.

BALANCED OIL SUPPLEMENTS

These are to be avoided. In 1986, Udo Erasmus in his book, *Good Fat-Bad Fat*, advised a balance of Omega 3s (fish oil), Omega 6s (polyunsaturated), and 9s (monounsaturated) fats. Today, most knowledgeable doctors discourage this practice. We do need essential fats, but we get enough Omega 6 in our regular diet because it is in almost all prepared foods. The monosaturates, such as olive oil, are neutral. If we consume the neutrals, we tend to consume less of the polysaturates, which are unhealthy.

Monounsaturated fats (monos) are considered neutral, but many have some other effects according to a 1999 article in the journal *Neurology*.[3] These oils (olive oil, in this case) decreased age-related cognitive decline or Alzheimer's disease. Compared to other vegetable oils (the polyunsaturates), the monos have no adverse effect on the lipid profile. The oil with the most monos is canola (rapeseed), but the most commonly used is olive oil. Cold-pressed extra-virgin oil is far better than other refined olive oils in that it also contains anthrocyanins. Walnut oil has recently been shown to have better health properties. These oils have a higher content of tocopheral and polyphenols. Compared to other processes of refinement, they reduce the susceptibility of LDL cholesterol to oxidation and vascular uptake (atherosclerosis).

Coconuts for the Brain

The brain uses mainly glucose for its fuel, but it works far better when it is fed ketones. Ketogenic diets have been used in medicine since 1924, initially to prevent seizures, and recently to treat degenerative neurologic diseases such as multiple sclerosis, ALS, stroke, and dementia. Thirty years ago, medium chain triglycerides (MCTs) were found to be metabolized into ketones by the liver. No longer did one have to eat the very stringent ketogenic diet, which was 70 percent fat, 25 percent protein, and only 5 percent carbs. A person could ingest a given amount of MCTs and produce their own ketones. Ketones do supply cerebral energy metabolism (provide alternative fuel), protect cerebral function, suppress cerebral edema, and reduce the extent of cerebral infarction in brain injury.

The presence of ketones in circulation, even at low levels, increases cerebral blood flow by as much as 40 percent. Ketones also prevent diseases involving free radical damage such as occurs in coronary reperfusion, diabetic small blood vessel disease, inflammatory bowel disease, and pancreatitis. MCTs do not behave like the more common long chain fats. Because of their shorter structure, they are metabolized directly in the liver into ketones rather than going into storage in fat cells. They are used as an alternative source of energy when glucose stores are exhausted.

Two years ago a drug company applied for and received a patent to bring out ketones as a prescriptive functional medical food. The Acerra Company brought out Axona to treat Alzheimer's disease.

The neurons work 30 percent better using ketones rather than the usual glucose. It is like putting high-test gas in an old high-compression engine; it runs much better, without the "pings." In a review article on Alzheimer's in the *New England Journal of Medicine*, the metabolism of the brain cell was detailed as "type 3 diabetes," in which the glucose receptors were blunted and could not transport the sugar into the brain cell to produce ATP for cellular energy. Not only could the cell take in the ketone, but it made ATP (energy) more efficiently. MCTs have been medically used in the past for feeding premature infants, for recovering surgical patients, and for malnutrition. Off label it has been used for liver support, antimicrobial therapy, enhancing the immune system, and increasing athletic performance. Contrary to popular opinion, these tropical saturate fatty acids inhibit atherosclerosis instead of producing it. They also decrease appetite and help people lose weight, much like the ketoses of the Atkins' Diet. Also there is not a tendency for diabetics to have problems of "diabetic coma," (keto-acidosis), with MCTs.

"Coconut oil" is a misnomer, in that it is solid at room temperature. It contains over 60 percent MCTs. Not only is this a healthy cooking oil in that it has a high smoke point, but it has a pleasant taste. It can be used in baking, oatmeal, spreads, and salad dressings. Costing $8 for 14 ounces for organic and $5 for regular, it is almost a best buy because this cooking oil doesn't smoke unless the temperature exceeds 280 degrees. Butter smokes/burns at a much lower temperature, producing free radicals that "rust" our bodies. Research at NIH by Richard Veech, MD, indicates that ketones that are made from coconut oil and MCTs work better since a higher dose is more easily achieved.

To treat Alzheimer's today and give a high dose of MCTs (20 grams per meal) to increase ketosis, you will need to combine 16 ounces of MCT oil with 12 ounces of coconut oil, and use seven teaspoons at a time. It should be stored at room temperature, and increased gradually from two teaspoons per meal up to seven. Giving too much at a time initially will cause abdominal cramps and diarrhea.

Although it costs twice as much, one can use Axona, which may be paid for by some insurance plans and certainly by flex plans. It has a pleasant coconut taste when used as a cold drink with a meal. There are no Omega 3s in this mixture; therefore I recommend some fish or fish oil during the day because this complements the MCTs for improved brain function. The APOE4 Alzheimer's responds better to this therapy, because the brain starts developing defects in glucose metabolism decades before the development of the disease. Those who have a strong family history for Alzheimer's or memory problems earlier in life might consider starting this treatment now! Coconut oil is also great to keep the skin more pliant and wrinkle free. In addition to taking it internally, rub it on your skin.

Ominous Omelette

Eggs have been vindicated in the last two decades as a villain causing cholesterol plaque buildup in our arteries. Is it true? Actually, it depends how they are cooked. It is true that egg yolks contain the highest amount of cholesterol of any other type of food, but it is also high in healthful micronutrients, such as choline for our brain and cysteine, the all-important building-blocks of protein formation. It is not the cholesterol we eat that is critical, but the cholesterol our body produces depending on our genetics and the other kinds of "foods" we eat. In an individual prone to develop high cholesterol and atherosclerosis, trans fats, sugars, and oxidized foods are culprits. The cholesterol in the egg is oxidized when cooked in ways that expose it to air and high heat. Therefore scrambled eggs and omelettes have a large amount of oxidized cholesterol, which clog up our blood vessels if we are genetically unfortunate—as is 30 percent of our population particularly the APOE4s. Egg *white* omelettes, however, are healthy.

ALE, APE, and AGE stand for Advanced Lipid End products, such as in egg yolks; Advanced Protein End products, which are found in roasted foods; and Advanced Glycosylated End products, such as in caramelized foods (cooked sugars). These are pro-oxidants that "rust" our arteries by oxidizing our body's cholesterol after production. Although they taste better than the non-oxidized portion, these delicious crunchy morsels are dangerous to our health in causing not only cardiovascular disease, but also cancer! In cooking any food, the hotter it is, the more dangerous it becomes. The worst method is grilled, followed by roasted, then baked, in which the food is heated up in excess of 212 degrees. Far better are poached, braised, boiled, and Crock-Pot methods. Because the water never exceeds 212 degrees in the preparation of these items, little or no ALE, APE, or AGE, and no oxidized cholesterol occurs. The three are absorbed into our bloodstream and directly impacts our artery walls.

Poached or boiled eggs, or maybe even a fried egg, are okay since the cholesterol-containing yolk remains intact. But even fried eggs have some APE; the delicious brown "skirt" around the white. It also has ALE from the butter or oil used in frying.

Coconut oil produces very litte ALE. This is why, in general, fried foods are not healthy. Antioxidants, which we should be consuming, do mitigate some of this. I now eat boiled or poached eggs, occasionally a fried one, rarely an omelette, and never a scrambled one! If you really want an omelette or scrambled egg, use egg substitute or egg whites.

Chocolate: Friend or Foe?

For several decades I've been interested in knowing if chocolate is anything more than a delicious, but fattening treat. There are over eighty chemicals in chocolate that have been shown to be beneficial to man. There are also some negative ones. The beneficial ones include minerals (particularly magnesium), vitamins (B6, niacin, thiamine, riboflavin), hormone-like chemicals (ferulic acid and phosphatidylcholine), stimulants (caffeine and theobromine), amino acids (threonine), pain relievers (nicotinamide), aspirin-like anti-platelet compounds, as well as several other chemicals that have antiseptic, anti-oxidant, and antiparasitic properties.

Chocolate comes from the cacao tree, a small evergreen that grows as high as twenty-five feet in the wild, but when cultivated is only five feet, convenient for hand-picking. One-inch-long, reddish-brown beans are imbedded in a white pulp. The chocolate nuts are taken from this, and after a simple fermenting process, such as burying them under leaves for several days, they are ready for use. In the New World chocolate was consumed in a bitter, spicy drink called xocoatl, and was often flavored with vanilla and chili pepper. Until the sixteenth century, no European had ever heard of the popular drink from Central and South America. It was not until the Spanish conquest of the Aztecs that chocolate was imported to Europe. The first chocolate house opened in London in 1657. In 1689, noted physician and collector Hans Sloane developed a milk chocolate drink in Jamaica that was initially used by apothecaries but sold to the Cadbury brothers in 1897.

Chocolate in its solid form was invented in 1847. Joseph Fry & Son discovered a way to mix some of the cocoa butter back into the dutched chocolate, then added sugar, creating a paste that could be molded. The result was the first modern chocolate bar.

One ounce of dark chocolate contains the same amount of antioxidants as a five-ounce glass of red wine. Even the fat in chocolate (cocoa butter), which was once thought to be bad, is now known to be mostly stearic acid, which is far better for our arteries than other saturated fats.

The smooth rich taste of chocolate has to do with palate-pleasing physical properties, as well as with almost 300 aromas and flavors to tease the taste buds and tweak the brain. Dark chocolate has far less fat and more of the "good stuff' than light chocolate. White chocolate has none of this. I would advise reading the label to make sure there are no hydrogenated oils, excessive sugar, or artificial flavors, which are sometimes used in less expensive forms of chocolate. Hopefully, xylitol (a sugar alcohol sweetener used as a naturally occurring sugar substitute found in the fibers of many fruits and vegetables) is used.

Chocolate has been shown to have positive benefits for human health. Panamanian Indians who consumed a cocoa-ladened drink (xocoatl) had one-third fewer incidence of cancer and cardiovascular disease. The first epidemiological study proved the more cocoa (chocolate) intake the better the cardiovascular system and a decrease of all-cause mortality; it took place in Holland. The Zutphen Elderly Study published several years ago in *The Archives of Internal Medicine* revealed that men who ate the most cocoa had a significant drop in blood pressure and a 50 percent lower risk of cardiovascular death.

In a more recent study of 44,489 people, those who ate one serving of chocolate per week had a 22 percent reduction in the likelihood of stroke. Another study found that people who ate fifty grams of chocolate each week were 46 percent less likely to die following a stroke.

The New Cholesterol

Most heart attacks occur in folks who have not only normal cholesterol, but decent levels of its subtypes, HDL (Healthy Dynamite Lipid) and LDL (Lousy Darn Lipid). Also, some who have elevated cholesterol and LDL with a low HDL have no cardiovascular disease. Oxidized LDL is really the villain. But more important, there is an advance lipid test that gives much better information. Three labs that do these include the VAP test (short for Vertical Atherogenic Profile), developed at the University of Alabama, Birmingham (UAB) Medical Center, and the LPP (Lipoprotein Particle Profile) test offered by SpectraCel Laboratories in Houston and The Cleveland Heart Laboratory. These are a boon for doctors and better for their patients who do not want to be just treated for heart disease, but rather prevent it before it happens. This is a reliable risk assessment in that we can now break down the components of cholesterol, and single out the most dangerous fractions.

Here are just a few of the key readings these tests give you that the old ones do not. Your LDLs were considered to increase the risk of heart attack and necessitate treatment. But LDL, for the most part, is really a good guy—a sheep slapped with a wolf's reputation. Your basic cholesterol is mostly LDL and wrapped in a protein coating (lipoprotein) that allows it to circulate in the bloodstream. Cholesterol is essential in the body for vitamin D, steroid hormones (like estrogen, progesterone, testosterone, and cortisol), bile acids, and as part of our cells' membranes. It also makes up 28 percent of our brain! LDL can be bad or good as identified by these tests. LDL becomes dangerous when it is oxidized or overly present as a small dense particle as opposed to a larger, fluffy more "buoyant" one (Pattern A). The small dense LDL is nefarious and is labeled Pattern B. B for Bad!! This is because the smaller BB-like particles are more easily able to penetrate the endothelium. There also is a determination of Intermediate Density Lipoprotein or IDL remnants. These can be incorporated into the arterial wall *without* the oxidation that the other lipids need to become atherogenic and considered extremely dangerous.

The tests also indicate a really bad type of LDL: Lp(a). This genetically endowed particle increases the risk of heart attack up to twenty-five times! It is highly inflammatory *and* thrombotic. There is no conventional medication for Lp(a), but niacin (vitamin B3), high-dose vitamin C with proline CoQ_{10} and N-acytel cysteine (NAC) may help. When using niacin beware that homocysteine, another risk factor in the blood, does not increase. It also raises blood sugar, uric acid, and liver enzymes which can cause heartburn and even eye problems. There is some controversy about long-acting non-flush niacin in that the wax or resin impregnated variety may cause more liver disease, but the long acting IHN (IsoHexoNiacinate) works very well. The dose of this vitamin must be high. I usually start at 3000 mg taken once a day and increase to 6000 mg to reach the goal. Because it is so helpful in all the other lipid disorders, this dose not only improves Lp(a), but lowers the LDL, raises the HDL-2, and converts the bad pattern B to the good A. It is cheap and does not require a prescription.

A high level of HDL—the so-called good cholesterol—is generally associated with protection against heart attack. We now know that HDL is further classified into HDL2 and HDL3. The difference between the two is that the active HDL2 is far superior to the inert HDL3 in providing protection for the heart. Triglycerides, which are incorporated in VLDL, are measured too, and anything above 100 (fasting) is considered abnormal. With these tests, the bad triglyceride (VLDL3) is singled out. This is the most inflammatory triglyceride, a cause for coronary artery disease progression, insulin resistance, and Type 2 diabetes. Triglycerides are fat globules in the bloodstream. In a concentrated form, they create abdominal fat.

The Advance Lipid Profile measures MPO and PLAC-2 both generators of unstable plaque. The former is decreased by acetomenaphen and the latter a drug will be forthcoming.

Protein

Protein is important because it provides amino acids, the building-blocks for all living tissue. It stimulates glucagon, a balancing hormone to insulin. Every day our bodies use and lose protein. Unlike fats and carbohydrates, protein from any source is protein, although some have more essential amino acids and may have a better balance of these molecules. Essential amino acids are those that our bodies can't produce, whereas our bodies can produce nonessential amino acids from any available protein.

Glucagon has the opposite action of insulin. It minimizes the adverse effects of too much insulin, which tends to make us fatter. The sources of all protein include fish, fowl, vegetables (legumes, whole grains), and meats. Non-animal sources are better than animal sources in that the methionine of the latter is converted in the body to homocysteine, which has been shown for the last three decades to be a significant risk factor in chronic disease.

Protein for Weight Loss

Diets concentrate, more or less, on fats and carbs such as the Pritikin/Ornish no-fat diet and the Atkins low carb/high fat diet. The Eades wrote about *Protein Power*, but others have cautioned that excess protein can be detrimental to the kidneys. When people with low kidney function eat more protein, there is decreased kidney blood flow and more protein in the urine.

In an article published in 1982 in the *New England Journal of Medicine*, Dr. J. Brenner showed this occurred in some, but not all, patients with *pre-existing kidney disease*. Twenty years later, Dr. Skov in Copenhagen noted this did not occur in *any* patients with normal kidney function. In a six-week trial with a high protein diet, there were no adverse kidney effects and no increase in albumin in the urine. MRIs and dopplers revealed as the kidney blood flow increased, so did the kidney size to compensate for this. This is similar to the enlargement of a muscle when it is exercised. In the Nurse's Health Study, those who had a high protein diet had lower cardiovascular disease. Several years ago, in the *Journal of the American Medical Association*, J. Obarzanek, MD, showed that high protein diets may be cardioprotective. Protein is good for weight loss in that it increases the metabolism and decreases the appetite. That is, it takes more processing to break down the protein for energy than fat or carbohydrates.

Protein switches on the genes that make the muscle protein actomyosin. This is particularly true in branch chain amino acids (isoleucine, leucine, and valine). These are found in higher concentrations in meat and fish, but not in vegetable proteins such as soy and legumes. They can be isolated and used to fortify products such as the "Workout Bar," for consumption prior to exercise to strengthen and improve muscles. Plant protein is higher in arginine than lysine. Arginine is associated with decreased cardiovascular disease because L-arginine is used by the body to produce nitric oxide, which is essential for cardiovascular health.

Not too many generations ago, hunter-gatherers, such as the American Indians, at times consumed up to 75 percent of their diet as protein. Buffalo meat has 84 percent protein and 16 percent fat. For lean health, a 50/50 balance of protein and the other half fat and carbs—but *no crap*—is advised. The protein should be of high biologic value. Of all the protein-rich foods, egg white has the highest value and quinoa is quite good. Fats should be mostly Omega 3s and carbs of a low glycemic index. The creator of the Paleo Diet, Dr. Loren Cordain, recently wrote *The Paleo Diet for Athletes*, which details this point of view.

Homocysteine Kills

The level of your blood homocysteine is associated with a higher incidence of mortality, including cardiovascular disease and cancer. Homocysteine is a natural amino acid that is toxic to our tissues in high levels. In 2003, the *New England Journal of Medicine* published back-to-back articles and an editorial that joined three other studies in denying this fact. In the first, an international randomized trial involved 5,600 patients with histories of documented vascular disease (peripheral, cerebrovascular, or coronary), or with diabetes plus another risk factor, who received supplements that had been touted to lower homocysteine: B12, B6, and folic acid. After five years, the average homocysteine level was 25 percent lower in the vitamin group than with the placebo, but there was no difference in cardiovascular deaths.

The other study involved a prevention trial from Norway where 3,700 patients who had recent heart attacks received the same B vitamins or a placebo. During an average follow-up of three years, the group receiving vitamin supplements had no decrease of repeat heart attacks. According to this, B supplements may lower the homocysteine, but they may not improve cardiovascular death among patients at high risk for vascular events. Researchers concluded that supplemental folic acid, B6, and B12 are not beneficial, and that homocysteine is merely a marker for other atherogenic factors and lowering this does nothing to help our cardiovascular health.

How can something that has been well established in the medical literature for almost twenty-five years suddenly be determined "inaccurate"? After I reviewed these articles, I felt that the prescribed dosage of B vitamins was too low. Second, they only lowered the homocysteine levels to 12 and not to the goal which, according to some experts, is below 7. It has been my personal practice to give enough of whatever is needed to obtain an ideal result. There are preparations that include 5mg of folic acid along with 50mg of B6 and B12 (which frequently is not absorbed and should be given by injection, although sublingually it works in some cases). However, if these do not work, I add the very inexpensive over-the-counter supplement betaine hydrochloride (TMG), which comes in a 635mg size (two with meals twice a day).

Occasionally I add riboflavin or SAM-e to the mix. At times, coffee or an underactive thyroid can contribute to high homocystine levels. The bottom line is to know what your homocysteine level is and if elevated, lower it to seven or below. In refractory cases, I use a thyroid supplement.

Vegetable protein, like all non-animal foods, has no cholesterol. Vegetables are also a good source of fiber, vitamins, and minerals. They can, however, contain a fair amount of carbohydrates. It is better to eat the leaves (lettuce, spinach), flowers (broccoli, cauliflower), and stems (asparagus, celery) than the fruits (plums, tomatoes) or the roots (potatoes, carrots), in order to limit carbohydrates. Legumes such as chickpeas or beans are also good sources of protein, but not soy. Grains such as quinoa are also great sources of protein.

Fish protein is rich in Omega 3 fatty acids (EPA and DHA). Fat from any source is calorie-dense, but this kind is full of healthy properties.

Fowl is also a good choice of protein; the white meat has less fat than the dark. As in all animal sources of protein, there is some non-harmful cholesterol, too. Beware—chicken factories may produce with arsenic used in their feed as an antiparisitic.

Red meats, including beef, pork, and lamb have protein, but the meat should be lean. We do not need to be concerned about the cholesterol in meat, but we should be aware of the possibility of hormones, pesticides and antibiotic accumulation. These are concentrated in the fat, which we should avoid anyway. Organic meat from grass-fed animals is best. The more the meat is cooked, the more fat is removed. Cooking it on a porous tray will help the fat drip out. Be aware that fat heated to over 215 degrees will burn, oxidize to ALE, and become harmful. Meat is an excellent source of many minerals such as potassium, iron, zinc, molybdenum, and magnesium, and it does contain some vitamins. Organ meats such as liver should be eaten minimally or not at all because they contain a lot of fat and purines that can raise uric acid.

L-ARGININE

In 1998, the Nobel Prize was awarded to Louis Ignarro for the discovery of EDRF (endothelium-derived relaxing factor), a chemical produced in the lining of the blood vessels, which keeps them healthy. Several years earlier, Dr. John Cooke, from Standord University and other investigators have found that specific nutrients can enhance EDRF production and improve blood flow in people with high cholesterol, high blood pressure, diabetes or other risk factors for heart disease. The atom of cardiovascular health—a tiny molecule called nitric oxide. NO, as it is known by chemists, is the signaling molecule produced by the body, a vasodilator that helps control blood flow to every part of the body.

Arginine, or more correctly L-Arginine, is the natural molecule in our body that produces NO in the one-cell-thick lining of our blood vessels called the endothelium. NO has a beneficial effect on the whole cardiovascular system. It relaxes and enlarges the blood vessels, prevents blood clots that trigger strokes and heart attacks, and regulates blood pressure and the accumulation of plaque in the blood vessels. Current research indicates that NO may help lower cholesterol by facilitating the actions of statin drugs like Lipitor or lower lipids by itself. It also has been shown to improve the immune system, facilitate healing, prevent cancer, enhance nerve and brain function, and act as an anti-aging molecule by stimulating HGH (Human Growth Hormone).

Arginine is a conditionally nonessential amino acid, meaning in healthy young folks it can be manufactured by the human body, and does not need to be obtained directly through the diet. *But* in older people or those with other diseases, including stress, the biosynthetic pathway does not produce sufficient amounts, and it must be consumed through diet. Arginine is found in a wide variety of foods, including red meat and dairy products. However, these need to be consumed in large quantities such as two pounds of steak or three quarts of milk daily. This so-called food is inflammatory and causes vascular disease and cancer.

In our bodies, Arginine is synthesized from another semi-essential amino acid, citrulline, by several cellular enzymes. But it is very energy costly; with each molecule produced two ATP equivalents are used up. In healthy humans, synthesis of Arginine occurs principally in the intestines and kidneys. The lining of the small intestine produces citrulline primarily from glutamine, which naturally is in our diet if we eat healthily. The kidney extracts citrulline from the circulation and converts it to Arginine, which is then returned to the circulation. Consequently, poor diet or impairment of small bowel or kidney function can reduce Arginine and NO. To make matters worse, there is a competing molecule that some of us have in our body, ADMA, which causes an even lower level of NO and health.

Since the early 1970s, L-Arginine has been used as a supplement with modest effects, but in the last five years there have been several good products available. Engineered by Dr. Ignarro himself are Niteworks and most recently Pro-Argi 9. These have at least 4 grams of L-Arginine, 200 mg of L-citrullene, and chaperone molecules such as vitamin C, folic acid, and alpha lipoic acid. It comes in a canister or packets of powdered product. One scoop or packet is taken at least ninety minutes after eating and immediately before sleep. Carbohydrates and protein inhibit its intestinal absorption, and when taken at bedtime it stimulates HGH release as well as insuring a good night's sleep. Certainly one could double and even *triple* the dose for better and quicker health benefits, but it is not necessary. There are less expensive sources of L-Arginine that may work just as well, but be sure to take an adequate dose.

Uric Acid

Two scientific premises have recently come together: "Lowering uric acid decreases death and aging," and "elevation of bile" does the same. An inexpensive drug, Probenecid, can improve both of these. In *JAMA*, researchers reviewed the literature showing that elevation of uric acid is not only a predictor of gout but is commonly present in new onset high blood pressure. Other previously documented research reports that elevation of uric acid contributes to cardiovascular disease, including stroke, heart attack, and peripheral vascular problems. Uric acid reduces nitric oxide levels in the lining of arteries, causing them to be more easily damaged. A well-controlled double-blind study on the lowering of uric acid using the drug Allopurinol resulted in a significant reduction of blood pressure. As noted in the past, hypertension is a significant risk factor in cardiovascular disease because of its role in atherosclerosis, stress to the heart, and acceleration of the inflammatory processes of the body.

Bile (bilirubin) was long considered merely a metabolic waste product from the breakdown of red blood cells discarded in the liver. Bile in the intestinal tract functions to markedly improve our fat digestion by emulsifying it. For the last twenty years, this pigment has been shown to decrease hardening of the arteries, prevent blood clotting, and reduce the risk of damage to the brain after a stroke. It has been recognized to have anti-inflammatory, antioxidant, and cyto-protective properties. The NHANES (National Health and Nutrition Examination Survey) is published every ten years by the U.S. government. It represents a cross-section of our national population; it has been carried on for fifty years involving over 13,000 patients each decade. According to this survey, those people who had higher bile had a marked decreased incidence of neurological damage due to stroke and, incidentally, they also had a decreased incidence of heart attack and peripheral vascular disease. The study was carefully controlled for other risk factors to include hypertension, diabetes, lipids, homocysteine, C-reactive protein, and body weight.

Those who had significant liver disease, a very common cause of very high bilirubin, were not included. However, it has been long noted that those folks with high bilirubin, for whatever reason, had far less hardening of the arteries. A rare benign inherited elevation of bilirubin disorder (Gilbert's Disease) has also been shown to have an increase of longevity. These findings are suggestive that elevation of bilirubin is an important defense mechanism against atherosclerosis, and it protects against neurologic injury in case of stroke. The well-tolerated Probenecid, as noted above, not only lowers uric acid but raises bilirubin.

A strategy for a decrease of vascular disease and all accrued benefits is to have your doctor prescribe Probenecid, 500 mg a day. This will raise the bilirubin slightly and significantly give anti-inflammatory and cyto-protective effects increasing longevity. Normal bilirubin levels are from 0.1 to 1.3, and if the bilirubin is between 1.1 and 2.0, you are much better off. People do not become jaundiced unless their bilirubin is over 3.0. A "home remedy" without using a doctor is to consume a fair amount of ox bile; this will also help lower uric acid levels to the ideal (less than 5). This will improve your lipids and your bowel and raise your bilirubin to protective levels. Although a double-blind study has yet to be done, it is almost a no-brainer to at least consider this healthy strategy.

I frequently prescribe the inexpensive generic allopurinol to lower uric acid in high-risk patients. I also avoid use of the antihypertensive diuretic hydrochlorathezide, the most commonly prescribed drug in the United States. It does raise uric acid, but it also depletes our bodies of magnesium, and it raises sugar and triglycerides.

No Joy in Soy

A decade ago I spoke of the joy in soy, but since then there have been as many negative articles about this once loved plant protein as there have been positive. In Israel, soy milk is substituted for real milk when meat is eaten because Jews still believe the Old Testament law, "Thou shalt not boil a kid in its mother's milk."

In conducting some original research and reviewing the world's literature, the Israelis concluded that soy should be used only in moderation. Soy contains trypsin inhibitors that decrease protein digestion and negatively affect pancreatic function. The phytic acid in soy reduces the absorption of iron, zinc, and calcium, and it increases the need for vitamin D. More significantly, soy contains isoflavones, which not only stimulate the growth of cancer cells, but they also decrease the effect of natural estrogens and thyroid on their respective receptors. They are considered *Hormone Disrupters*. Soy also widens the pubertal age gap between boys and girls. With the use of soy, girls mature as early as age eight while boys do so at fourteen.

As a food, soy dates back several thousand years. It was only after the Chinese learned to ferment soy to make foods like tempeh, natto, and tamari that it became edible. It has been mistakenly thought that Asians eat a large amount of soy and that it prevents cancer of the prostate and breast in this ethnic group. Actually the consumption of plain soy in Asia is minimal. It is fermented and used as a condiment rather than a replacement for animal protein.

Even the protein in soy is not complete. Like all legumes, soy is deficient in methionine and cystine. Modern processing denatures the fragile amino acid, lysine. Studies showing that soy reduces cholesterol and benefits heart disease are outweighed by the increase of heart disease through the reduction of vitamin D. It functions in almost every cellular process in the body and may, in itself, prevent heart disease because of its effect on lipid and sugar metabolism. Free glutamic acid and MSG, both potent neurotoxins, are also formed during soy processing, and additional amounts are frequently added to soy foods. Soy is high in aluminum, which is shown to be toxic to the nervous system (causing Alzheimer's) and the kidneys.

Soy blocks the normal surge of testosterone production in the first six months of life. The long-term ramifications of this has much to do with sexual determinates and even cancer. Two decades ago, when a marked disparity of breast cancer in the United States was compared to that of Japan, it was thought that soy products were actually protective in preventing breast cancer in Japanese women. However, later studies showed that this may not be so. Actually, it is the much lower fat in the diet and decreased alcohol intake that makes the difference.

In addition, a quarter of the population has a subtle allergy to soy that can produce symptoms ranging from brain fog to migraine headaches, as well as common allergies such as stuffy nose, itchy eyes and hay fever.

Carbohydrates

Carbohydrates are sugars and starches found in vegetables, legumes, grain (starch), fruit (simple sugars), dairy (dis-accharides), refined sugars, and flour from any source. They should be consumed in moderation because carbohydrates stimulate insulin production from the pancreas. There is a direct correlation between how much and how quickly carbohydrates are eaten and how much insulin is released. Insulin itself is not bad, but it is dangerous in excess amounts. If it is not balanced by glucagon, it elevates blood pressure, causes atherosclerosis, produces bad eicosanoids (a type of hormone), decreases the ability to concentrate, and makes us fat. Insulin causes hunger and places our most recent food consumption directly into our fat cells unless we exercise right after eating. Most Type 2 diabetics produce too much insulin and carbs are implicated.

Glucagon, another hormone produced by the pancreas mainly when we eat protein, neutralizes the adverse effect sof insulin. Thus, it is important to eat as much protein as carbohydrates. Some nutritionists recommend eating protein before eating carbohydrates. Excess carbohydrate consumption causes water production and, water retention since these are metabolized into carbon dioxide and water.

One needs to consider the total amount of calories, as well as the glycemic index of the food (see below). If you consistently eat calorie-dense foods, especially containing fat, it certainly will add to your already fattened body. With extra insulin, fat goes right into the fat cell; whereas if carbohydrates change to fat, calories are burned in the process and fewer calories go to fat.

GLYCEMIC INDEX (GI)

The glycemic index (GI) was first developed in 1981 by a team of scientists led by Dr. David Jenkins, then at the University of Toronto, to help determine which foods were best for folks with diabetes. At that time, the diet for diabetics was based on a system of carbohydrate exchanges. It was too complex to be easily taught to patients.

Eating low on the GI enhances memory and cognition, helps weight loss, lowers blood sugar, decreases triglycerides, increases energy, and prevents vascular disease. It is a physiological fact that glucose stimulates pancreatic insulin release. The faster and the higher glucose is released in the digestive tract, the more insulin will be released in the blood. This is modulated by naturally produced incretins such as amylin. Insulin is a two-edged sword. Beneficially, it is needed to drive sugar into the cells, but if too much glucose (and subsequently, too much insulin) is in our system, it can have a damaging effect, causing high blood pressure, adverse lipids, increase of arteriosclerosis, and worst of all to our vanity, *obesity*. Food is energy, but if that energy cannot be used immediately, it is initially stored as glycogen in the liver and, subsequently, into the adipose cell as *fat*.

Food is ranked on a scale from 0 to 100, with glucose having the index of 100. The higher the index, the more insulin is released from the pancreas and the more fat is produced to be stored. Table sugar (sucrose) has a GI of 65. Fructose alone has a GI of 53. Starches have the highest GI, with a potato having 100! On the other hand, white bread has 72; stone ground whole wheat has 53. Pastas are not nearly as bad, with spaghetti having a GI of only 41. White rice has a GI of 72 but Uncle Ben's Converted Rice is 44. Dried dates are 100; apples, 38; oranges, 44; grapefruit, 25; and cherries, 22. The less ripe the fruit, the better. Green-yellow bananas are

Table 3-VIII
GLYCEMIC INDEX

The higher the Glycemic Index, the more insulin the food will produce. Eating foods lower on the Glycemic Index will encourage weight loss by lowering the insulin level.

High Inducers of Insulin (Bad)

Grain-based foods (GI>100)	Grain based foods (GI 80-100)	Vegetables
Puffed rice	Grapenuts	Carrots
Corn flakes	Whole-wheat bread	Parsnips
Puffed wheat	Rolled oats	Corn
Millet	Oat bran	**Fruits**
Instant rice	White bread	Bananas
Instant potatoes	Instant mashed	Raisins
Microwave popcorn	potatoes	Apricots
French bread	White rice	Papaya
Simple Sugars	Brown rice	Mango
Maltose	Muesli	**Snacks**
Glucose	Shredded wheat	Tofu ice cream
		Puffed rice cakes
		Ice cream
		Corn chips
		Rice crisps

Moderate Inducers of Insulin (Better)

Grain-based foods (GI>50-80)	Fruits	Simple sugars
Spaghetti (white)	Orange	Lactose
Spaghetti (whole wheat)	Orange juice	Sucrose
Pasta, other	**Vegetables**	**Snacks**
Pumpernickel bread	Peas	Candy bars
All-bran cereal	Pinto beans	Potato chips (with fat)
	Garbanzo beans	
	Kidney beans	
	Baked beans	

Reduced Insulin Secretors (Good)

Grain-based foods (GI 30-50)	Applesauce	Kidney beans (dried)
Barley	Pears	Lima beans
Oatmeal	Grapes	Tomato soup
(slow cooking)	Peaches	**Dairy products**
Whole-grain rye bread	**Vegetables**	Yogurt
Fruits	Peas	Ice cream (high fat)
Apples	Lentils	Milk (skim)
Apple juice	Black-eyed peas	Milk (whole)
	Chick-peas	

Lowest Insulin Inducers (Best)

Fruits (GI <30)	Simple sugars	Snacks
Cherries	Fructose	peanuts
Plums	**Vegetables**	
Grapefruit	Soy beans	

better than brown-yellow bananas, and Granny Smith green apples are better than red ones. Parboiling or not overcooking decreases the GI. The starch, which is stored in a protein packet, is broken up by cooking, increasing the GI. Thus, al dente pasta (firm to the bite) will have a lower GI. A carbohydrate with a GI greater than 50 is referred to as a crapohydrate.

Chana dal, chickpeas, and the wonder food, quinoa, are tasty, versatile, and healthy, with a GI of less than 25. Low GI foods are filling. Physically eating slowly lowers the glycemic index in that the food goes into the intestines less rapidly, with less production of insulin. Adding lemon juice or vinegar will tend to lower the GI of all foods. These acids decrease the stomach's emptying rate. Adding lemon juice or vinegar to part of the salad dressing works well. Consuming a mixture of high and low glycemic foods together results in an intermediate GI. Some nutritionists refer to the glycemic load, which takes into consideration not the weight but the serving size of a particular food. See page 147 for a more detailed listing.

Don't Be Simple; Be Complex

A simple vegetarian will consume simple carbohydrates (sugars and starches) and the products that contain these fattening, non-nutritional ingredients like bread, pasta, and white rice. There is a world of complex carbohydrates out there that are recommended for health, not just for religious or animal rights purposes.

Second only to cricifer sprouts beans, to include Chana Dal (page 160), but not soybeans, lead the list of a nearly perfect food. These are high in complex carbohydrates, amino acids, soluble and insoluble fiber, vitamins, and minerals. Although bean protein is considered incomplete because it is low in methionine, it will transform into a complete protein if you eat nuts, grains or whey periodically. Beans are packed with phytochemicals, which are anti-cancer as well as anti-

PHYTOCHEMICALS:
What they do and which foods have them?

Phytochemical	Possible Action	Food Source
Allicin. allylic sulfides	Induce emeymatic detoxification systems; may act against *Helicobacter pylori;* allylic sulfides may reduce BP and cholesterol levels.	Onions, garlic, scallions, leeks and chives.
Capsaicin	Neutralizes carcinogenic benzopyrenes/substance P.	Chili peppers
Catichins	Reduce cholesterol levels preventing oxidation; inhibit phase I and II enzyme systems, which plays a role in carcinogen activation.	Green tea, straw berries, raspberries and other berries.
Chlorogenic acid	Blocks formation of carcinogenic nitrosamines	Tomatoes, green peppers,pineapples.
Flavonoids (4,000 different compounds, including flavonols, isoflavones, and flavones)	Antioxidants; reduce cell proliferation; increase the pump-mediated efflux of certain carcinogens from cells; isoflavones inhibit bone resorption.	Widely distributed in fruits, vegetables, wine, tea.
Indoles	Spur enzymes to form an estrogen; thought to be protective against breast, colon, esophageal, prostrate and lung cancers.	Cabbage, broccoli, Brussels sprouts, cauliflower, kale collards, mustard greens, turnips and rutabaga.
Limonoids	Increase production of protective enzymes	Citrus fruits, particularly the rind.
Monoterpenes	Antioxidants	Broccoli, cabbage, citrus fruits, cucumbers, eggplant, parsley, peppers, squash, tomatoes and yams.
P-Coumnaric acid	Blocks production of cancer-causing nitrosamines	Tomatoes, green peppers,pineapple and strawberries.
Protease inhibitors	Lengthen the time it takes for cancer cells to develop.	Soybeans, cereals and beans.
Triterenoids	Suppress carcinogenic activity of estrogen.	Soybeans, licorice root extract, citrus fruits and carrots.

fat nutrients. White Northern beans and others contain pha-soleum, a natural starch blocker. Undercooked, crunchy beans have oligosacchrides, a gas-producing chemical that causes them to be "musical," but which feeds our good intestinal bacteria. Fully presoaking and cooking the beans can prevent this. Except for split beans (garbanzos, chana dal, and peas), beans should be soaked for twelve to thirty-six hours and the discarded water used to make plants healthier.

When cooking, do not boil beans furiously, as they will burst and thus denature their healthful contents. Dry beans last a year. Cooked, they last five days in the fridge or six months in the freezer.

Even healthier than cooked beans are sprouted beans, seeds, and grains. Sprouts are a fresh mini-harvest. See the details below. They are energized with live enzymes, including the anti-aging SOD (superoxide dismutase). Sprouted beans and grains have increased vitamins. The best sprout is broccoli, which provides fifty times the amount of cancer-protective glucosinolate as mature broccoli. Whole grains, nuts, and beans are part of a healthy diet. To enhance the flavor of these, add sea vegetables. These can be purchased in most health food stores and include arame, dulse, kombu, and wakame. They contain fantastic protein as well as Omega 3s! Going easy on fruits and fruit juice is recommended because they contain a high amount of simple sugars.

BROCCOLI IS HEALTHY, BUT THEIR SPROUTS ARE BETTER

Edible sprouts are germinated plant seeds. They are usually produced by soaking the seeds at regular intervals over a four to ten day interval. *Broccoli* sprouts are highly nutritious, with magnesium and chlorophyll. They are rich in enzymes and electrons that promote good health as mitochondrial en-hancers and antioxidants. Studies of compounds in broccoli sprouts have been shown to reduce the risk of prostate, breast, liver, stomach, bladder and colon cancer, and acts as an antibacterial agent against Helicobacter pylori, an organism associated with causing duodenal ulcers. Also, broccoli sprouts decrease the risk of stroke, high blood pressure, and cardiovascular disease, as well as osteoarthritis.

Research has shown that broccoli sprouts are rich in glucoraphanin, a compound that when eaten is converted in our body into *sulforaphane* (sul-FOR-a-fane) glucosinolate, which is a "phase II inducer." In 1997, Paul Talalay, PhD, who founded the Brassica Chemoprotection Laboratory at Johns Hopkins, identified chemoprotective nutrients and found ways to maximize their effects. Also in a study funded by the British Heart Foundation it was discovered that sulforaphane could "switch on" a protective protein that is inactive in parts of the arteries vulnerable to plaque formation. Scientists already know that arteries don't clog up in a uniform way, but that there are bends and branches of blood vessels in which blood flow is disrupted (turbulence) and are much more prone to the build-up of fatty plaques that cause heart disease. In the more vulnerable areas, a normally protective protein known as Nrf2 is inactive. Sulforaphane protects those regions by switching on the Nrf2.

Brassica is a plant in the genus of the mustard family and in addition to broccoli, it includes brussel sprouts, cabbage, kale, cauliflower, and turnips. Three-day-old broccoli sprouts contains more than a forty times higher concentration of the protective molecule than mature broccoli. In addition, cooking destroys three-quarters of the active compound. Eating a few tablespoons of these sprouts daily can supply the same degree of cancer and vascular protection as twenty pounds of *cooked* broccoli eaten weekly.

Broccoli sprouts can be frequently obtained at health food stores or in concentrated juices or capsules, but they may not be as good as producing this fantastic food yourself and eating them fresh. The seed and sprouting trays are easily obtained and the growing initiated by soaking four tablespoons in a eight-ounce jar of water overnight (about eight hours). Pour the soaked seeds onto the sprouting tray. These trays and the organic seeds can be purchased at most health food stores and online at websites such as the Sproutman.com. Cover the tray so the enclosure provides a greenhouse effect. Rinse by showering the seeds with fresh water twice per day. Try not to dislodge the seeds with the force of the rinse water. Allow the seedlings to root themselves into the small holes of the growing tray. Keep the tray away from strong light for the first four days, then move to a brighter area, avoiding direct sunlight and heat. In three to four more days they will be green and ready to harvest. Pluck from the surface to allow the younger sprouts to continue to grow. In the next three days, they should all be sprouted. With prayer and luck, you should have two pounds of health from them. They can be used in cooking and in sauces, but they are healthier used as salads or in sandwiches made with red cabbage leaves or kale rather than bread. Do yourself a healthy favor and you will be rewarded well beyond the minimal work it takes to eat this wonderful delicacy that will add life onto your years and years onto your life!

EAT LIKE A KING

Your grandmother knew that you should have a good breakfast. This has been proven in a double blind study published recently. People who eat a higher proportion of their daily food early in the morning have a significantly lower caloric intake the rest of the day than those who eat little or nothing during the morning hours. The study included almost 1,000 individuals who completed a detailed food diary in a weeklong study. Individuals who ate with the participant verified the accuracy of their report. Meal size increased throughout the day and intervals decreased between meals in those who had minimal morning intake. Those individuals were less satisfied by each successive meal as the day progressed. Meals eaten during the morning produced the greatest satiety, while meals eaten in the evening produced the least.

The bottom line is: The greater proportion of food consumed during the morning hours, the lower the total intake and conversely. Eating no breakfast and a large meal late in the day was associated with a marked total increase of calories and the tendency for obesity. Therefore, one should eat breakfast for a king, lunch like a prince, and supper like a pauper. It certainly makes sense to fill up your gas tank before you start an automobile trip rather than after you get to your destination. Food eaten after 6 p.m. when physical energy is low, or at night when physical expenditure is minimal, causes the caloric content to be deposited in our fat reservoir rather than burned as fuel. In our modern society, many folks skip breakfast or eat minimally, but most consume the worst of all caloric intake, carbohydrates (such as doughnuts), in the morning or the so-called healthy cereals that are advertised to kids.

The human body is not made to use much carbs, but rather to consume protein and fat, which are used for building of our tissue; what is left over is burned for energy. On the other hand, when you consume carbs, if they are not converted into energy immediately, they are stored as fat for subsequent use. Therefore, over the millennia we have evolved to consume protein and fat rather than carbs. Moreover, in the past, it was survival of the fattest rather than the fittest, but now in the land of plenty (where there are carbs, and particularly crapohydrates, galore), we are producing an epidemic of obesity.

Mushrooms

Mushrooms have been favored for centuries, not only as food, but also as remedies against aging. According to some practitioners, the Reishi mushroom has been used clinically against cancer, cardiovascular disease, chronic fatigue syndrome, hepatitis, herpes, hypertension, high cholesterol, HIV, and for weight loss. The Shiitake, a first cousin to the Reishi and Japan's largest agricultural export, has been used as a remedy for upper respiratory disease, poor circulation, and fatigue. It may also prevent premature aging. Today, however, it is recognized most for its immunologic activity and as an anti-tumor agent. The Maitaki, also from Japan, has been advocated to strengthen the body and improve overall health. These are giant mushrooms, often twenty inches in diameter; a single cluster can weigh up to one hundred pounds. Recently they have also been used against hepatitis, cancer, HIV, and for regulating blood pressure and blood sugar. Aside from the medical benefits, mushrooms taste good, are low in calories, are very filling and are not too costly. There are some expensive ones, such as Gama Derma, which reputedly produce even higher levels of immunity. A whole host of other mushrooms are reputed to improve health with particular attention to cancer and infections such as Lyme disease.

FIBER

Fiber is important because it cleans our digestive system like a good scrub brush and diminishes such diseases as cancer, diabetes, diverticuloses (itis), gallstones, hemorrhoids, and even appendicitis. Regarding cancer, its preventive effectiveness is unclear. A recent study shows that fiber did not have any effect on colon cancer. According to the 1999 *American Journal of Gastroenerology*, it is low animal product consumption that is beneficial, not fiber. The method of defecation can also affect gastrointestinal diseases. Going only when necessary and squatting over, rather than sitting on, a toilet with three-inch blocks under the feet and squeezing the upper calves is recommended.

Fiber can be soluble or insoluble. It is a non-absorbable

carbohydrate and therefore contributes no calories unless there is a mismatch of "Good (Bacteroidetees) and Bad (Firmiculties)" bacteria in the colon. Then, there is a breakdown of fiber to simple carbohydrates and production of a chemical that rapidly transforms the carbs into fat for storage. Probiotics improve this situation. More about this when we discuss our wonderful friends whom we allow to reside in our gut. The best fiber, which really is a prebiotic, is amylose resistant corn starch and Fibersol-2, which causes an increase of the fat-reducing bacteroidetes who inhabit our colons.

Chana-Dal Beans

Chana-Dal is not a doll from China, but a legume: a bean inside a pod that splits in two. It is a close cousin to both garbanzo beans (chickpeas) and lentils. The wonderful fact about Chana-Dal is that it has a glycemic index of only eight! That means, for one serving, it takes more calories to consume and digest this food than the calories gained from eating it. However, if one eats too much at a time (three or four servings), it can cause bloating, gas, and diarrhea.

This is an ancient food that became famous in Indian literature. Historically, 400 years ago, the king of the Taj Mahal was taken hostage by his estranged son, who turned against and later overpowered the Taj. He could not kill his own flesh and blood, so he exiled the king to another castle that can still be seen from the Taj Mahal. He told his distraught father that he could take only one food for his imprisonment, but he could also take his personal chef. The son told the father to be careful which food he chose, because that was the only food he would eat for the rest of his life. After consulting with his chef, word was sent to the king's son; the food would be Chana-Dal. The cook had told the king he could have a new dish every day for the rest of his life, no matter how many decades that would be.

You can experiment or use these beans when recipes call for either garbanzo or lentils. These beans are used in large amounts in Indian and Oriental cultures. They can be purchased from almost any Asian or Indian grocery store or delicatessen in larger cities.

Since Chana-Dal has nondigestible carbohydrates in the form of fiber, it will improve bowel function and may prevent many diseases of the intestine we have in the twenty-first century, such as diverticulosis, appendicitis, colon polyps, and even cancer. Should the excess fiber cause any problems with gas, a few drops of Beano, bought at any health food store and used on the first few spoons during the first few weeks, will aid the situation.

Following is a sample recipe to get you started:

Chana-Dal—Simple

Soak 1/2 cup of beans in water overnight. In the morning, drain off the water, put seasoning of choice on it, and eat it cold; or place in a microwave for 40 seconds and eat hot. Your favorite seasoning or spice will make it taste better, whether it be sweet (add xylitol) or salty (add a salt substitute).

THE WONDER FOOD: QUINOA

As many as 10 percent of us have gluten intolerance, and quinoa (*keen-wah*) is a storehouse of wonderful nutrition and can be used as a wheat substitute. It has 2 grams of magnesium, 6 of protein, and 3 of fiber in a quarter cup! Quinoa is a grain-like crop grown primarily for its edible seeds. It is a pseudocereal rather than a true cereal or grain, as it is not a grass. As a chenopod, quinoa is closely related to species such as beets and spinach. Its leaves are also eaten as a leafy vegetable, much like amaranth, but the commercial availability of quinoa greens is currently limited.

Quinoa was of great nutritional importance in Andes mountain civilizations for over 5,000 years. Locally referred to as "Mother Grain," secondary only to the potato and followed in importance by corn, it kept the Incan armies strong and robust. In contemporary times this crop has become highly appreciated for its nutritional value, as its protein content is very high (12 to 18 percent), making it a healthy choice for vegetarians and gluten intolerants. Unlike wheat or rice (which are low in lysine), quinoa contains a balanced set of essential amino acids for humans, making it an unusually complete protein source, almost as complete as the milk protein casein. Lysine is one of eight essential amino acids—building-blocks of protein—that the body cannot manufacture on its own. As a building-block of protein, lysine benefits the body by contributing to growth in babies and children. Lysine benefits also include production of carnitine, a substance that converts fatty acids into energy and lowers levels of LDL cholesterol.

In addition, lysine benefits the skeletal system by contributing to the production of collagen, the protein used to make bone, tendons, cartilage, and connective tissue. Calcium absorption is also facilitated by lysine, and lysine benefits the skin by helping to maintain its health and elasticity.

Quinoa is easy to digest and is ideal for the first "grain cereal" given to infants. Many doctors feel giving oats, wheat, and barley to infants sets them up for a lifelong allergy problem. Because of all the above characteristics, quinoa is recommended by the Food and Agriculture Committee of the United Nations for underdeveloped countries and is being considered a possible crop in NASA's Controlled Ecological Life Support System for long-duration manned spaceflights.

Raw quinoa has a sapin coating that is irritating to the digestive tract, causing gas, cramps, and diarrhea, and must be washed off before consumption. Most boxed quinoa has been pre-rinsed and some even sprouted for convenience. Sprouting any grain by leaving it at room temperature for a given period of time enhances its healthy attributes. Quinoa may be germinated in its raw form to boost its nutritional value by leaving it in water for only two hours at room temperature. Wheat takes twelve hours! Germination activates its natural enzymes and multiplies its vitamin content.

A common cooking method is to treat quinoa much like rice, bringing two cups of water to a boil with one cup of grain, covering at a low simmer and cooking for fourteen to eighteen minutes or until the germ separates from the seed. The cooked germ looks like a tiny curl and should have a slight hardness to it (like al dente pasta). As an alternative, one can use a rice cooker to prepare quinoa, treating it just like white rice (for both cooking cycle and water amounts). Vegetables and seasonings can also be added to make a wide range of dishes. Chicken or vegetable stock can be substituted for water during cooking, adding flavor. It is also suited to vegetable pilafs, complementing greens like kale and spinach. Quinoa can be added to salads and other cold foods to enhance filling of the stomach and give a health boost. Quinoa can serve as a high-protein breakfast food mixed with xylitol, almond, or berries. It is also sold as a dry product, much like cornflakes. Quinoa flour can be used in wheat-based and gluten-free baking. For the latter, it can be combined with sorghum flour, tapioca, and potato starch to create a nutritious gluten-free baking mix. A suggested mix is three parts quinoa flour, three parts sorghum flour, two parts potato starch, and one part tapioca starch.

This powerhouse nutritional product is available at some avant-garde grocery stores and is available at most health food shops. "PEARL QUINOA—Soul Food of the Andes" has recently been promoted by ALTER ECO, a Bolivian co-op that is democratically managed by its farmers for sustainable development with profits used for organic programs. This is the product that I use. Quinoa comes in easily sealed bags for about

$8 per pound. For all those interested in their own health and the health of their loved ones, I recommend this gluten-free, nutritious, and versatile health food.

Vinegar for Vigor

Vinegar was discovered accidentally over 15,000 years ago. Since then, it has enriched man's life by not only preserving foods but also affording better health. Some of its health benefits have been proven in recent years. When taken before a meal, it moderates the appetite and decreases the glycemic index of high carbohydrate foods. In many cases of "ulcer pain" and heartburn, which is caused by *not enough* stomach acid, a warm cup of diluted vinegar alleviates the problem. Nocturnal leg cramps, urinary tract infections, acid-based imbalance, constipation, diarrhea, and infections can be "cured" by drinking this miraculous fluid.

The sting of a Portuguese man-of-war (a jellyfish) can cause nausea, headache, chills, and even cardiovascular collapse. Some of these effects can also be mitigated by applying vinegar. Venom from insects can also be alleviated by a dab of vinegar.

The American Academy of Otolaryngology endorses the use of vinegar and alcohol to prevent and treat "swimmers' ear." This inflammation of the external ear canal is due to the growth of fungus or bacteria. Simply dilute vinegar half and half with boiled water and, for a more drying solution, mix that with an equal part of alcohol. Applying vinegar to the skin encourages the normal acidity of the tissue. It is used as a compress for many skin conditions.

Bacteria and fungus (athlete's foot, vaginal yeast infections) as well as dandruff are discouraged by vinegar. It kills odoriferous underarm bacteria and hence can be used as a deodorant and is good for sunburn. It makes insoluble minerals, such as the very inexpensive magnesium oxide and calcium carbonate, soluble to be more readily absorbed by our intestines. When used on food, it tenderizes meats and vegetables, enhances the taste, and kills the lethal E Coli bacteria.

Used as a sterilizing agent, vinegar kills germs and insects when fresh fruits and vegetables are dipped into vinegar water. Rubbing it on wood cutting boards not only kills the bacteria, but also cuts the grease and absorbs odors.

There is a host of other uses for vinegar, including decreasing the static electricity and lint on clothing, making them sparkle when taken from the dryer. It also reduces buildup of minerals on plumbing fixtures, stops mold, and cleans eyeglasses, window glass, and metal. For these uses, inexpensive vinegar (less than $1 a quart) helps, but for our health, organic, cloudy apple cider vinegar is best.

All vinegars are not created equal. Although the healthiest is organic apple cider vinegar, many fruits can make this wonderful liquid. Beware of commercial products that could be made out of sulfite waste from paper mills and petrochemicals. These have the 5 percent acetic acid but none of the wonderful, healthful properties of natural vinegar. It lacks the amazing MOTHER of vinegar; chain-like strands of protein enzyme molecules that mysteriously produce this magic elixir. Our ancestors used vinegar to improve the taste and particularly for the preservation of food. Prior to the advent of refrigeration, salting, drying, and sugaring would prolong the "shelf life" of food. Marinated (soaked in vinegar) or fermented foods would last for decades and enable man to survive times of famine. Today, we do have pickles and sauerkraut made with vinegar that is subsequently pasteurized (sterilized), killing the healthy MOTHER.

Vinegar was a fortuitous finding by our ancestors who, similar to their modern counterparts, liked to drink alcohol. Alcohol is made by the first fermentation of plant carbohydrates (sugars and starches), but a second fermentation turns this alcohol into a better product—vinegar. In fact, the word *vinegar* comes from the French term *vin* for "wine" and *aigre* for "sour." There are at least four types of live organisms that make this wonderful MOTHER from carbohydrates.

Apple cider vinegar is not artificially filtered, heated, or pasteurized and is diluted with purified water to 5 percent acidity. The brown color is from the healthy apple tannins and prevents oxidation of organs and body tissues.

In addition to the most prevalent acetic, vinegar contains lactic, propionic, and isobutyric acid. Moreover, there are dozens of enzymes, amino acids, and minerals, including potassium, magnesium, iron, and silicon in the natural product.

Commercially prepared vinegars are, unfortunately, pasteurized and filtered, killing the healthy MOTHER and destroying the natural healthy materials within. Good brands such as Braggs vinegar, produced by Drs. Patricia and Paul Braggs, is aged in wood and is one of the healthiest, costing less than $5 a quart. MOTHER is seen floating within the cloudy brew and is the sign of a continuing life.

The Doctor in the Fridge

There has been much in the medical literature about pH. Specifically, pH stands for the potential of hydrogen and is an indication of how acidic or alkaline a solution, or in our case, our liquid body is. It is measured on a logrythmic scale from 1 to 14. A pH of 7 is considered neutral. Anything less than 7 is acid and greater than 7 is alkaline. The further away the number is from 7, the more acid or alkaline is the fluid.

Vinegar (acetic acid) has a pH of 3, seawater of 8, and baking soda greater than 10. Since we as mammals came from the ocean, our tissue pH is slightly greater than 7. Our blood and fluid between the cells normally has a pH of 7.34 to 7.4, with our intracellular pH slightly lower. Maintaining the pH within this ideal narrow range keeps our metabolic machinery and immunologic defense systems working better.

There are three main systems that help keep the pH normal: the respiratory (lungs), the renal (kidneys), and our several buffering systems (specific neutralizing molecules). If these are working well and we do not throw in an excess load of acid or alkaline, our body stays within the healthy normal range of pH. Deviating from that, particularly to an acid state from aging, stressors, toxicity, and the impropriety of our modern diet, there could be an increase of cancer, infection, and other degenerative diseases such as arthritis and atherosclerosis.

Most fruits and vegetables contain a higher portion of alkaline-forming elements than other foods. On the other hand, some are acid forming, such as commercial corn, grains, and soybeans. This may reflect breeding selections in the last fifty years that favor a higher fat and carbohydrate content. Meats are acid formers.

Organically and biodynamically grown forms of grains and grasses are much less acid forming. Despite their pronounced acidic taste, citrus fruits and particularly lemon and lime, form higher alkaline metabolites. This is because their distinctive organic acids, such as citric, succinic, fumaric, and malic, are chemicals produced in the metabolic energy pathway termed the Krebs Cycle. This metabolizes carbs to water and bicarbonate, while producing energy inside the cell. Foods including chocolate, alcohol, coffee, and almost all meats, fish, poultry, eggs, and milk products are metabolized to acid by other pathways.

Our acid and alkaline state, as measured by the pH, varies throughout the day depending on when and what we ate. An inexpensive pH paper strip to test our value is available at hardware and health food stores to check our acid and alkaline balance. There is a normal diurnal variation with the highest pH occurring in the latter part of the day, particularly after eating a high fruit diet and the lowest, the first thing in the morning. Although salivary pH can be checked (first thing in the morning before drinking water or brushing the teeth), it is easier to check a urinary pH. A few drops of urine are placed on a pH test strip and referred to a color chart where the pH can be easily read. If the pH is lower than 6.5 in the morning, a change in diet is recommended. If your pH is not what you want and lifestyle changes don't fix it, consider baking soda. Baking soda is not baking powder, which has starch added.

I recommend taking one half to one teaspoon baking soda in a glass of water twice a day, once in the morning and once before bedtime. I also recommend adding a few drops of concentrated lemon juice in warm water twice a day. Even more healthful, but much more expensive, is a mixture of sodium, potassium, and magnesium bicarbonate. If you use this method, check the pH periodically to make sure it is not higher than eight and watch your blood pressure so that the sodium in the sodium bicarbonate does not raise it. If your blood pressure is regularly high, decreasing the amount of bicarbonate would be my recommendation rather than stopping it altogether. Most people will begin to feel better within twenty-four hours. Folks notice a decrease in stiffness and fatigue almost immediately and as the years go on, a decrease of infection, cancer, and other degenerative diseases.

Baking soda is a useful and healthful way to combat the ravages of modern society, where we have drastically strayed from the previously healthful paleolithic lifestyle of our ancestors. Today we also have much more toxicity in our environment, as well as stress from a continual time crunch. There are many expensive products that will help raise the pH, including herbs, but the "doctor in the refrigerator"—baking soda—is more efficient and much more economical.Also consider Kangen water, as noted earlier in the book. Not only is it alkaline, but is full of electrons and is microclustered for ease of entry into our cells.

FIRE IN THE HOLE

One could classify hot sauce, the spicy kind, not the elevated temperature of a heated sauce, as a food or herb, but we will discuss this under "food" because the main ingredient is the pepper. Since the days of Columbus, peppers have been used to flavor and preserve both meats and vegetables: the hotter the pepper, the less bacteria will grow. The heat in peppers is measured scientifically in Scoville Heat Units. Wilkes Scoville was a pharmacologist who, in 1912, developed the method of quantifying the "heat" in a pepper. The mildest bell pepper has zero units, sometimes referred to as heat units or RU, while habañeros rate three hundred thousand units. Incidentally, mace has only two hundred thousand units. Even a mild bell pepper grown twenty yards away from a cayenne can claim some Scoville Heat potential. The hottest are chipotle regular and the habañero (Scotchbonnet pepper).

The active ingredient in hot peppers is *capsaicin*, which, as many pain sufferers know, can be rubbed on an inflamed body part bringing much relief, although the first time or two, it will burn the skin. Capsaicin, which now is available as a prescriptive patch, antagonizes the action of substance P, the neurotransmitter or chemical that activates the neuron (nerve cell) that transfers the message from a pain site to the brain. In addition to blocking pain, capsaicin stimulates circulation, aids digestion, and, as those of us who have used hot peppers know, promotes sweating. Because perspiration works to cool the body, cayenne is sometimes used to break a fever. Post-operative pain, cluster headaches, shingles, and aching muscles are other occasions to use capsaicin.

An occasion, however, is hardly necessary. Tabasco sauce has been around since 1868, when the McIlhenny family of Louisiana developed their formula. Today it is a standard condiment in most homes and restaurants. I have recently begun placing three to four drops of Tabasco in my coffee for a better, spicy taste and alertness. Similarly, salsa is now served to schoolchildren, who also eat Tabasco-flavored jelly beans. (I eat a spicy salsa many mornings for the capsaisin, lycopenes [from tomatoes], and garlic added for taste.) Considered by some as simply flavor enhancers or salt substitutes, these sauces have also been credited with decongesting nasal passages, boosting the metabolism, enhancing the immune system, and even extending life. In addition to the hot peppers, these sauces may include other ingredients such as vinegar, salt, or mustard seeds.

If the sauce has fruits or vegetables in it, refrigerate after opening unless it will be consumed within a month. Unfortunately, the sauces are not rated according to Scoville Heat Units but with the subjective descriptors "mild," "medium hot," and "hot." There are many variations of each, but the names may provide a clue: "Cape Fear," "Hellter and Damnation," "Capital Punishment," and "Screaming Sphincter." All, especially the last, warn of fire in the hole. Contrary to popular belief, these fiery peppers themselves do not cause ulcers, although some folks may be intolerant and/or unaccustomed to their spiciness. Most problems come instead from the food on which the sauce is placed. Antidotes for the heat include yogurt and adding lemon or vinegar to the mixture before eating it.

Fruits

Fruits are another cancer- and age-fighting food. However, most fruits are high in the glycemic index. (However, cherries and berries are not.) These are high in antioxidants. Choose from the common strawberry to the exotic Acai berry. I also suggest eating grapefruit or drinking its juice daily. It makes certain drugs, such as statins (for lowering cholesterol), calcium antagonists, anti-hypertensives, digoxin, and non-steroidal anti-inflammatory drugs somewhat more powerful by increasing their activation. Grapefruit has a glycemic index of only thirty-six, and naringenin, one of its active substances, may also speed up our metabolism. Similarly, its limonoid (see chart IV-6) helps the immune system detoxify carcinogenic compounds. One large grapefruit or a glass of juice may last the body all day. This might be why grapefruit is the cornerstone of the Mayo Clinic Diet for weight loss. The content of limonoid and naringenin varies among juice types and brands. Fresh ruby red grapefruit contains the most. One can discount the calories in this fruit, which comes from its high carbohydrate content since it increases caloric burn-off. Of course, this assumes no sugar. If you want sweetness, add xylitol. Stay away from dried fruits like cranberries, dates, figs, and pineapples. Not only do they have a high glycemic index, but they are frequently laced with sugars.

WINE IS FINE

In my mind, there is not much controversy regarding the benefits of alcohol, particularly red wine. This is not to say that I recommend it for everyone. Certainly, if there is pregnancy, an addictive personality, seizures, liver disease, a strong family history of alcoholism, age less than twenty-one, or for religious or ethical reasons, I would not advise this healthy liquid. That being said, 70 percent of adult Americans can and should drink alcohol moderately. Moderation is no more than two drinks a day and a four-hour window before one does detailed mental or physical work or puts oneself in harm's way by climbing ladders or operating motorized equipment. Alcohol has been recommended for health since man first learned how to ferment fruits and vegetables. It was given a healthful quality, as noted biblically: "Use a little wine for the sake of your stomach and your frequent ailments" (1 Timothy 5:23). Thomas Jefferson was a very intelligent and "conservative liberal" who stated: "My diet is that of fruits and vegetables, a rare meat dish, and one drink a day. I have one and a half drinks with a friend and occasionally drink twice that when I am involved with "self-joy."

The Framingham Study, ongoing research detailing twenty-five years of alcohol consumption, has shown that alcohol is cardio-protective. When this information was made available, the U.S. government at the time was Republican and a little far to the right. The information was squelched. In 1985, however, our government finally announced that alcohol, particularly wine, decreased the incidence of coronary artery disease. In 1995, the *Nurses Health Study*, which had been going on for thirty years, officially recommended drinking as good for health unless there was a contraindication. Studies indicate that women who drink wine in moderation generally weigh less than those who do not.

There are some naysayers concerned that people who drank more than two drinks a day had a higher incidence of hemorrhagic stroke. However, most strokes are due to de-creased blood flow and clotting rather than hemorrhage. In fact, there are thirty times more strokes due to this than hemorrhage.

Over the last decade, information has come out on the benefits of alcohol for one's health. It does decrease the severity of diabetes, the incidence of heart failure, stroke, coronary artery disease, and Alzheimer's disease. With wine, particularly red wine, the polyphenol component has been shown to decrease the risk and rapidity of many cancers. More than three drinks a day, however, increases the risk of breast cancer by 4 to 6 percent in women. Drinking significantly more than that increases the incidence of cancer to as much as 400 percent!

If one were to chart on a graph life expectancy with the number of drinks per day, those who do not drink will die earlier than those who drink in moderation. According to some studies, drinking 1.7 drinks a day decreases the incidence of coronary artery disease by 35 percent. With wine, one can increase that to two and a half glasses a day. With more than that, there is a steady increase in all causes of mortality: commonly, accidents, cancer, and hemorrhagic strokes. High alcohol consumption does take its toll on society with personal failures impacting occupations, relationships, and families.

It has been shown that alcohol improves the level of the good cholesterol (HDL), slightly decreases the bad cholesterol (LDL), and decreases the very bad oxidized LDL cholesterol, which forms plaque. The HDL (High Density Lipoprotein) cholesterol, which has some antioxidant activity, improves reverse cholesterol transport. In addition, alcohol decreases the platelet (small elements in the blood that cause clotting) stickiness, increases the dissolution of clots, improves sugar metabolism, and decreases nitric oxide destruction. Nitric oxide causes vasodilatation and offers protection from atherosclerosis.

The dark color of wine is from phenolic compounds in the grape skin, making it reddish and cardio-protective. However, the effect lasts only twenty-four hours. Therefore, for this benefit, one must drink red wine on a daily basis; the darker the wine, such as pinot noir and red zinfandel, the better. Wine also contains resveratrol, which turns on the SIR2 longevity gene. The grape with the most resveratrol is the Sangiovese, from which we get chianti wine.

Again, I do not routinely recommend alcohol, and if I did, I would particularly advise red wine. As mentioned earlier, if you have liver disease, seizures, pregnancy, an addictive personality, a strong family history of alcoholism, an age of less than twenty-one, religious prohibitions, or if you need your brain and reflexes to remain at peak performance, you should not drink.

Health Is As Easy as A-B-C

A-B-C stands for Acidophilus-Bifido-Certified live yogurt.

Yogurt can be not only low in calories and fat, but contains probiotics that are the real secret to its biggest health benefits. The live cultures in yogurt create its creamy texture and sour taste as well as a healthy intestine. These bacteria are called *probiotics*, a term that means "for life" and refers to any live organism in food that has benefits beyond simple nutrition. Probiotics are showing up in all sorts of health food drinks and supplements, though yogurt is still their main source.

The two key bacteria in regular yogurt are *streptococcus thermophilus* and *lactobacillus bulgaricus*. Their work is to turn milk into yogurt by gorging on the milk's sugar (lactose) and converting it to lactic acid. The lactic acid works the proteins into such knots that the whole solution curdles. This fermentation allows even people with lactose intolerance to eat this dairy product. Yogurt bacteria contain their own lactase, which goes to work on any milk sugar that is left over from fermentation. When these bacteria hit the small intestine, digestive juices split them open, releasing enough lactase to break down the milk.

A variety of *lactobacillus* (l. bulgaris, l. hamnosus, l. acidophilus, l. casein), *bifidobacterium* or bifido (b. bifidum, b. longum, b. zinfantis) are added to the culture. Researchers have been aware of bifido since the early 1900s, but few strains survive well in yogurt. Unlike other bacteria, which are killed by stomach acids, these strains wade past the stomach and settle in the small and large intestines. They manage to thrive in the intestine's balanced ecosystem of other benign and beneficial bacteria.

When this equilibrium is upset by harmful food-borne bacteria, like salmonella or campylobacter, diarrhea frequently results. Acidophilus and bifido may help suppress such an infection by crowding spaces where damaging bacteria would otherwise attach themselves and by releasing acids that destroy the invading germs. Reseeding the intestine with these beneficial microbes can also stem diarrhea and other side effects of some antibiotics. Because antibiotics are indiscriminate in their wrath, killing good bacteria along with the bad, at the end of a course a person may have a seriously depleted intestine. Acidophilus and bifido also tip the balance of the thin/fat ratio to decrease fat loss. Eating yogurt along the way can control the damage.

Acidophilus yogurt may combat vaginal yeast infections as well. In a 1992 study of women with recurrent infections, those who ate eight ounces of acidophilus-rich yogurt daily for six months had significantly fewer infections than in the previous six months. They also fared better than women who ate no yogurt at all.

Probiotics may also fuel the immune system in a more generalized way. A study showed that yogurt with acidophilus appeared to increase the activity of phagocytes, the white blood cells that destroy invading germs. Other studies suggest bifido might be a cancer fighter. Research has shown that eating yogurt containing bifido bacteria switched off an enzyme associated with colon cancer.

Because many commercial products have fewer probiotics than homemade yogurt, I recommend you make it yourself. Just buy a starter package from a health food store and follow the directions on the label, or ask a healthy friend to give you four ounces of his or her already prepared yogurt. You can also begin with a health food store brand of live acidophilus yogurt that is specifically labeled as such and add Hi-Maise corn starch and b. rahamnogus. Using a home yogurt maker with an automatic incubator is an easy way to make this health food. Each time I make yogurt, I save four ounces with which to begin the next batch. I have known families who brought their yogurt culture from overseas decades ago and still use it. There are a few healthy products that are made individually in plastic containers (look for a healthy plastic number on the bottom). They have at least six different probiotics, are gluten free and use pectin rather than starch as a thickener. One with national distribution is Activ8 (found at *www.cascadefresh.com*). Better, as noted below, is a better probiotic choice, along with its own food, *prebiotics*. Together they are called synbiotics.

Probiotics—Our Friend Within

Probiotics are live microorganisms that, when administered in adequate amounts, confer a health benefit on the host. Our intestines have been populated with friendly bacteria since birth. We carry, as an adult, eight pounds of this biomass. It is another independent living organ inside of us that has evolved with us since ancient times. Periodically, to maintain a healthy environment after digestive problems, and certainly after taking antibiotics, I recommend replanting our gut with probiotics. These are a live culture of both bacteria and yeast. They are dedicated not only to discouraging unfriendly organisms from taking up residence in our gut, but proper pH, gas production, and stool consistency, with a decreasing incidence of intestinal diseases is the result. These diseases include peptic ulcer (caused by a hostile bacteria: H. pylori), "colitis," gallbladder disease, colon cancer, and a whole host of nonintestinal problems such as hypertension, vitamin K production, hyperlipidemia, diabetes, osteoporosis, obesity, poor immunity, and urogenital disease. They also produce signaling chemicals that go to our liver and improve or worsen our body structure and function, such as acne and rosacea in our skin. Antibiotics wipe out dozens of species and end up making us less healthy in the long run.

Composition of an individual's gut micro-flora is a recently recognized factor in diet-related obesity. Two groups of the bacterial phylum of micro-flora are dominant in the human gut, the Bacteroidetes and the Firmicutes. The relative proportion of Bacteroidetes is decreased in obese people by comparison with lean people, and that proportion increases with weight loss. An obese phenotype has been associated with a relative abundance of the bacterial phylum Firmicutes, resulting in increased "energy harvest" or caloric extraction from the diet. Firmicutes are predominantly Clostridium, but include Lactobacillus, some of which are in the probiotics we unknowingly recommend. In terms of effects on intestinal carbohydrate- and lipid-digesting enzymes, it has been shown if the population of Firmicutes outnumbers Bacteroidetes, partially digested complex carbohydrates are broken down rather than eliminated through the stool. These, then, form simple sugars that are easily absorbed in the bloodstream. A special chemical is elaborated by this bacterial digestion. This encourages the sugar to be directly made into triglycerides by the liver and preferentially stored by fat cells rather than burned. Additionally the certain strains within the Bacteroidetes produce a lipid-digesting enzyme. The net result of having more Bacteroidetes and less Firmicutes is a decrease "energy harvest" or caloric extraction from the diet and a loss of 100 calories a day, which represents twelve pounds a year just by having the right ratio of the B/F. There have been some specific bacteria of the Bacteroidetes group such as *Lactobacillus rhamnosus* PL60, which produces conjugated linoleic acid and in itself has anti-obesity effects. The combination of pre- and probiotics, known as synbiotics, has been proposed to characterize some functional foods with interesting nutritional properties that make these compounds candidates for a weight loss program. One such is high-amylase-resistant cornstarch laced with *Lactobacillus rhamnosus* PL60 and other Bacteroidetes species. Some scientists have even proposed to rid the gut of most of the Firmicutes with Xifaxan and then repopulate with Bacteroidetes.

It is by no accident that we have these two opposing groups of bacteria. With famines, these floral reverse ratios were life-savers, but in modern times, with too much food and too little activity, they are a killer. Therefore, a high B/F ratio causes weight loss and a low ratio weight gain. Some scientists have proposed that high frutcose corn syrup is a prebiotic for the Firmicutes group, thus favoring the spread of this fattening factor to modern humankind. This adds insult to injury to the high empty carb load for more fat gain.

Combining probiotics and prebiotics in what has been called a symbiotic. They beneficially affect the host By improving survival and implantation of beneficial species. By selectively stimulating the growth or activating the catabolism of one or a limited number of health-promoting bacteria in the intestinal tract, the gastrointestinal tract's microbial balance upgraded. Combining probiotics with prebiotics could improve the survival of the bacteria crossing the upper part of the gastrointestinal tract, thus enhancing their effects in the large bowel. Moreover, probiotic and prebiotic effects might be additive or even synergistic. This has been the case when combining the anticarcinogenic effects of the prebiotic, inulin.

Flax Facts

Flax, a tall, leafy-stemmed plant with shiny blue or white flowers contains flat golden or brown seeds that are full of nutrients. It now grows wild in many areas of the United States, although 100 years ago it was cultivated just as it was in ancient times. Woven flax cloth has been found in Egyptian tombs and, from Hippocrates on, flax has been used medicinally. Decades ago it was used as glue, as homemade hair gel, and as paint (linseed) oil. Recently, flax has been shown to assist memory, boost cerebral function, support the body's inflammatory response, and help with women's reproductive organs.

Flax contains essential fatty acids, soluble and insoluble fiber, proteins, vitamins, lignans, and other phytonutrients.

Flax oil is an abundant source of alpha-linolenic acid, which is converted to the healthy Omega 3s in our bodies only if we are young and healthy. It has a powerful cardiovascular effect, not only lowering total cholesterol and triglycerides, but also raising the HDL cholesterol. Moreover, Omega 3s decrease the coagulation of blood and may prevent heart attacks and strokes. Flax seeds contain ten grams of fiber in one-quarter cup. Fiber acts as a broom, cleaning out the intestines, not only promoting regularity but decreasing the incidence of colonic polyps, cancer, diverticulosis, and diverticulitis. More than that, lignans support our immune systems. These are low-glycemic carbohydrates.

I recommend two tablespoons or more of ground flax a day. It is safe for everyone, but because of its mild laxative effect, it may bother some folks with irritable bowel syndrome. Allergies to this health food are almost unknown. Golden whole flaxseed is inexpensive and may have slightly more nutrient value. Foods that contain whole seeds, like cereals such as Uncle Sam's, do little good for our health. It is far better to buy ground seeds or, better yet, whole flax seed and grind them in an inexpensive coffee grinder. Ground flax meal should be consumed within a day or refrigerated in an air-tight opaque container where it will keep for several months. When it spoils, it smells like paint oil.

Flax meal has a sweet nutty flavor and tastes delicious sprinkled over cereals, soups, and salads, or when used for baking in casseroles and breads. Ground flax mixes easily with juices. I do not recommend the use of flax seed oil, which is available in liquid or capsules. It is high in calories, and for most of us, it does not convert to the active Omega 3 oil in that the enzyme to work this magic is diminished in most of us. Not only is it more expensive and less palatable than flax meal, but it does not have the fiber, phytonutrients, or lignans found in the whole seed preparation. Ground flax meal is not to be eaten plain since it will firmly cake on the roof of the mouth and can be difficult to remove.

Go "Nuts"

Peanuts and peanut oil are monosaturated. The oil has not come into its own as a preventive to cardiovascular disease as has olive oil. Commercially made peanut butter can be hydrogenated, contain the bad trans-saturated fatty acids, and may include gluten. Also the samonella contamination of early 2009 makes it even more hazardous. Making natural peanut butter from peanuts is healthier. Although some people consider peanuts to be nuts, they really are not! Peanuts are legumes and grow underground. Until the early 1900s, they were referred to as goober peas.

Some seeds, such as sesame, sunflower, and pumpkin seeds, have wonderfully healthy oil. Even tiny mustard seeds have recently been touted to lower triglycerides and elevate the good HDL cholesterol. With all these one can buy or make natural seed butter or its milk. Be careful if you buy seed milk or butter that it is not loaded with high glycemic sweeteners.

An editorial in a recent peer-reviewed medical journal was titled "You Have to Be Nuts Not to Eat Nuts." Nuts and seeds also contain the beneficial gamma vitamin E, rather than the nonessential alpha vitamin E found in multi-vitamins and additives in so-called healthy foods.

Nuts contain abundant nutrients in addition to being a good source of plant protein (10 to 25 percent) and unsaturated fatty acids (50 to 75 percent). Their nutrients include vitamins such as folic acid, niacin, vitamin E, and vitamin B6; minerals such as copper, magnesium, and potassium; dietary fiber and phenolic antioxidants and phytosterols.

Four major epidemiological studies credit nut consumption with a 37 percent lower risk for coronary heart disease for those who consumed four or more servings per week, compared with those who seldom or never ate nuts. They noted a reduction of 8.3 percent for each incremental serving of nuts consumed per week.

FEELING YOUR OATS

Rolled oats, which have been softened by steam and flattened by rollers to form flakes, are the most common type of oatmeal. In contrast, steel-cut oats are small round nuggets. They do take longer to cook, but because of their hardy, chewy texture, they are much in demand and therefore more expensive. There is essentially no difference in the taste but the fiber and nutrient content of rolled oats is not quite as good as steel-cut oats. It is far better to use old-fashioned oats that have the husk on them (and more fiber) than "quick" or "instant" oats. Oats are caloric and acid-producing, but they are a healthier grain than wheat. Unless stated "gluten free," oats are contaminated with wheat and gluten. It is a boon to the nutritional community that coffeehouses such as Starbucks which now serves oatmeal as an alternative to the cookies and cakes that were their usual fare.

SAY NO TO GMO (MODIFIED FOODS)

A genetically modified organism (GMO) is a life form whose genetic material has been altered using recombinant DNA technology, with the nuclear material from different sources to create a new set of genes. The new organism then has a modified or even a novel set of genes. These are non-affectionately called "Frankenfoods." For conventionally grown fruit (grown with chemical fertilizers and pesticides), the PLU code on the sticker consists of four numbers: Organically grown fruit has a five-numeral PLU prefaced by the number 9. Genetically modified (GMO) fruit has a five-numeral PLU prefaced by the number 8. For example, a conventionally grown banana would have a PLU of 4011, but an organic banana would have a PLU of 94011. A

GMO banana would have a PLU of 84011. The numeric system was developed by the Produce Electronic Identification Board, an affiliate of the Produce Marketing Association, a Newark, Delaware–based trade group for the produce industry. "We hate eight, but nine is fine!" is the motto to follow. However, no store ever uses the number 8, since most folks would avoid GMOs if they were so labeled.

The benefits of genetic modification, however, are as persuasive as the drawbacks. Plants are engineered to be more resistant to cold weather and pests, and to require shorter growing seasons and use less fertilizer. This same technology can also create nutritionally power-packed plants called functional foods: fruits and vegetables that deliver more vitamins; nuts, milk, and cereals that are allergy free; plant "toothbrushes" that contain a chemical to prevent decay; plant oils with more Omega 3s; and food with increased macronutrients.

The adhesive used to attach the stickers is considered food-grade but the stickers themselves are not. There is a trend now to individually shrink-wrap the product which may not be so healthy because some of the plasticizer could migrate into the product. Hopefully this will be changed in the future. The best is to grow your own organic produce, or buy it from a farmer who does.

The Champagne of Fermented Foods

Kiefer is a functional food that has benefits beyond its basic macronutients. Although kiefer has been around since shortly after the Stone Age and was mentioned in the writings of Marco Polo, it wasn't until the early 1900s that Russia rediscovered this wonderful, healthful food. After the Cold War, it was given by Russia to the super powers in a symbolic gift exchange. Kiefer is a fermented milk product that, in the past, was produced by adding cauliflower-looking granules to milk. It is a tart, refreshing, effervescent drink enjoyed the world over by many millions, but very few here in America. It is yogurt-like, but much healthier. The consistency is slightly thicker than milk and unlike homogenized milk, is shown to produce atherosclerosis and other degenerative diseases. Kiefer decreases the incidence of these because the lactose is broken down to galactose, it is extremely well-tolerated by folks who have lactose intolerance. It has a dual fermentation, with both lactic acid–producing bacteria and yeast which produces minute amounts of alcohol, which help keep this material sterile. It is high in calcium, amino acids, B vitamins (including folic acid), vitamin K, biotin, pantothenic acid, and microorganisms. These produce specific antibiotic substances that control undesirable germs, which could cause disease such as infections and even cancer. One of the products in kiefer is tryptophan, which causes relaxation and improvement of many neurologic disorders such as depression, ADHD, and chronic fatigue. The principal beneficial metabolite in kiefer is a water-soluble product known as kieferan, which stimulates the immune system and regulates cholesterol.

It can be drank, eaten, used as a creamy base for dressings and sauces, or used in the making of milkshakes and ice cream. The finished product is available commercially as a slightly sweetened, flavored drink, but this is hard to find. Once made, kiefer can be kept in the cupboard rather than the refrigerator.

Kiefer can be found in most health food stores as inexpensive, freeze-dried granules. Hermetically sealed, they will last a lifetime with further home culturing. Along with the granules are simple instructions for home production and recipes for its use.

A Bridge over Troubled Waters

Good, old-fashioned water, the universal solvent, should be the bulk of any extra liquid intake. Accounting for 70 percent of the cells' weight, it provides the environment that makes life possible. We are "bioengineered" around the special properties of water. Its polarity, ability to form hydrogen bonds and surface tension regulate the free flow of water into our cells. In the human body, water resides in two molecular states—bound and transiently clustered. Bound water is physically attached to other molecules and is more restricted from moving through our cell walls. As we age, the quantity of bound water increases.

Water coming from deep subterranean wells and the polar ice caps has a greater proportion of micro-clustered water molecules. Soon after exposure to our environment, it reverts to the normal larger clusters, which are more difficult for the process of tissue transfer. Chlorine, an oxidizing agent added to "purify" our drinking water, injures the body. Several decades ago, Joseph Fisher, MD, discovered that chlorinated water promotes cancer and arteriosclerosis. His studies were suppressed by the water industry and therefore are not commonly known. Just letting plain tap water sit in an open container for several hours will remove much of the dangerous chlorine.

Running the tap for a minute to get rid of the first quart may decrease the contamination from the plumbing in the faucet, which has more potential harmful effects per inch than plain pipes. One of the harmful byproducts of chlorinated tap water is trihalomethanes (THMs), known to be carcinogenic and abortive. A prominent environmental group reported that they found fecal coliform bacteria in 1,172 water systems nationwide, lead in 2,551 systems, and radioactive materials (such as radon) in 326 systems. Other studies show that at least 43 percent of all water supplies violate federal standards and as many as nine hundred people a year in the United States die from waterborne diseases, such as cyrtospordium. MTBE, a gasoline additive, may cause cancer and has been found in thousands of water supplies. I recommend drinking water that's been "decontaminated" by reverse osmosis or by distillation. A good silver impregnated charcoal filter on the faucet may be an alternative. Also of interest, a coffeemaker's paper filter and grounds will markedly decrease the heavy metals in the water when coffee is brewed. In municipal cities, you can gain more information by calling the Safe Drinking Water Hotline at 800-426-4791, or you can visit the website www.epa.gov/safewaterinfo.htm.

Another choice may be some of the bottled water that falls under the jurisdiction of the FDA, which is less strict than the EPA standards for tap water. Some of these waters, which may be from springs, wells, or lake water, undergo purification by ozonization, reverse osmosis, a special "one-micron absolute filtration," and/or a special charcoal filter. These processes supposedly take out not only the impurities, but the disease-causing organisms. The taste of these waters varies, not only from their source, but also the material in which they are bottled. Those that come in PET plastic bottles generally taste better than the water that comes in HDPE. Do not reuse plastic bottles or leave them out in the sun where they could heat up. When the water is being shipped on pallets, we have no way of knowing if, or how long, they were left in the sun. Look for those that have a resistant plasticizer by the numbers on the container bottom. The plastics can leach into the liquid and act as hormone deregulators and even promote cancer. Some waters contain natural minerals, such as natural spring water costing thirty cents for eight ounces with no off taste. Others have the minerals, particularly magnesium, added back, such as found in Sam's Choice for six cents a serving. The better waters are in glass containers.

Water is naturally found in a lattice cluster formation with dozens of its sister molecules. The bigger the cluster, the more inefficient that water is in hydrating our individual cells. Kangen water does have microclusters and in addition, lots of electrons and can be made on the alkaline side for better health. Small cluster water results in a "wetter" water with better transportation of these molecules through the "pores" of our cells, carrying both oxygen and nutrients more efficiently. Vitamins, healthy chemicals, and herbal supplements are added to the water. Many special and expensive waters with their costly manufacturing processes such as alkanized, oxygenated, and ionically charged are available. One product is Microhydrin, which is taken as a capsule to make our internal water more "soluble."

We drink far too much water. Do the "eight glasses" math: 8 times 8 ounces per glass equals 64 ounces, or 1.89 liters. This amount of water alone is more than the total daily replacement needs for the average adult. And this is just drinking water that we're talking about. Solid food contains water, too. A cucumber contains about a cup of water; a medium peach, two-thirds of a cup. Even a dry piece of toast, when metabolized, creates one molecule of CO_2 and two of water. After adding up all of the water from beverages, water concealed in solid food, and water derived from invisible metabolic oxidation, one ends up getting much more than the daily requirement. And this is exactly what most Americans have been doing for several decades: consuming two to three times more water then they need. At the present time, the average daily water consumption by men in the United States stands at 3.7 liters (125 ounces, or almost a gallon), and 2.7 liters by women. In other countries water is used only in cooking and bathing, not for drinking. Do they know something that we Americans do not?

Be aware, however, if you have diarrhea, vomiting, fever, or heavy sweating from humidity and physical exertion. One has to make up for that by drinking more fluids. There is also a minute amount lost in our every breath. But in general, unless we are sick, are very active, or it is very hot, we do not need more than two glasses a day. There are six disadvantages to overdrinking water: It dilutes intestinal enzymes; it overworks our heart and kidneys; it decreases the concentrations of essential blood minerals; it increases the time and frequency of urination; it leads to excessive loss of minerals in urination; and it diverts our attention from the task at hand from when the urge comes until we urinate.

So why, despite the obvious facts and common knowledge, do grandmothers and most medical authorities think so very differently and urge people to drink more and not less? Because this is their teaching and it is not right. So hold on to your toilet seat and sit tight on your new knowledge. Leave the water under the bridge and cross over to dry land!

COFFEE FOR ME

For the past fifty years I have reviewed study after study of the pros and cons of drinking coffee. Some research implicates caffeine as the major con, and some point to coffee itself. Regarding caffeine, some who have a defect in caffeine metabolism experience cardiac arrhythmias (irregular and rapid heartbeats) from this chemical; others feel nervous and jittery during the day and are unable to sleep at night. Dr. James Lane at Duke University published that drinking five cups of regular coffee a day boosted the blood pressure of volunteers by five points compared to the days they drank just one cup. The pressure remained elevated for twelve hours. The author speculated that over the decades this slight increase of blood pressure could take its toll in premature cardiovascular disease. More bad news came from research showing that coffee elevates homocysteine in the blood. This significantly raises the risk of coronary artery disease, stroke, and all causes of death. Fortunately, paper coffee filters mitigate most of these harmful effects. In a study published in the *American Journal of Nutrition* in 2000, the unfiltered brew elevated the homocysteine level by 20 percent in a month, compared to when the same individuals drank filtered coffee eight weeks later.[4] Paper filters remove the diterpenes in the coffee that both elevate homocysteine and increase cholesterol production. It made no difference whether the coffee was decaffeinated or not. Coffee, compared to green tea, is acidic. Thus, if one must drink coffee, I recommend moderate consumption (one to three cups a day) using a double paper filter and made with Kangen water.

Coffee does have some health benefits too. The grounds remove 85 percent of heavy metals (lead, copper, mercury, cadmium, and zinc) from tap water. They may also capture other heavy metals.

Coffee will *prevent* type 2 diabetes according to a 2010 University of Oklahoma study, which found that people who drank *twelve* cups a day had a 67 percent lower risk of developing the disease compared to non-coffee drinkers. There was a more modest risk decrease for those who drank less.

Coffee may prevent or decrease gallstones, rheumatoid arthritis, migraine headaches, overhydration, Alzheimer's, and Parkinson's. It increases caloric burn during exercise if consumed right before a workout. Lastly, there is no definite evidence that coffee causes cancer. The healthiest part of coffee is the wonderful aroma, which lasts a few minutes after it is brewed. There is more of this polyphenol in the coffee if brewed with Kangen water. Therefore, brew by the cup and drink immediately, but *not* from a Styrofoam cup.

Take Tea and See

All teas, be they black, green, or white, come from the leaves of the same plant, Camellia sinensis. However, where the plant is grown, the amount of sunshine and water the plant receives, and the soil condition makes a vast difference in the quality of the tea. The color depends on which process is used in the drying and fermentation of the leaf. The more fertile the soil, the more amino acids are in the tea. The more sunlight, the more these are converted to antioxidants. The younger the plant the more expensive, but these have a higher amount of catechins and amino acids, particularly L-theanine.

The antioxidants, especially EGCG (EpiGalliCatechln-3 Gallate), help our immune system and have been shown in many studies to decrease the incidence of cancer and infection as well as relaxing our arteries. The antioxidant activity of EGCG is 100 times more potent than vitamins E and C. Black has the least, green more, and white tea the most of these micronutrients. One cup of green tea has an antioxidant activity greater than a serving of broccoli, spinach, or strawberries. The amount of the L-theanine is 15 to 30 mg per cup. Its benefits are improved healing and reduced stress. The L-theanine increases the production of the brain neurotransmitters serotonin and dopamine. These enhance mood and promote calmness and alertness. The dopamine also may decrease dementia and Parkinson's disease in older age.

L-theanine increases brain alpha waves, which lower blood pressure, heart rate, skipped heartbeats, and jitteriness. These are the same waves that are produced during meditation if done properly.

Tea does contain caffeine, but only 15 mg, compared to 100 mg per cup of coffee. In tea, the caffeine is neurologically neutralized by the L-theanine. Many people who drink coffee cannot do so with tea after noon because caffeine's effect on the brain keeps them awake at night. In addition, the xanthine in the coffee acts as a diuretic. This does not happen with tea.

If you are particularly sensitive to caffeine, however, you can buy the decaffeinated variety, or take more L-theanine as a supplement. This can be obtained at health food stores. Two hundred milligrams one to three times a day is recommended. Also, green tea extract can be obtained at these same stores. The drinking of a wonderfully healthy beverage, either socially or ritually, enhances its salubrious benefits.

Alcohol

As we have noted in our discussion of wine, alcohol may be consumed, but it is a double-edged sword. Too much of it impairs thinking and motor skills, decreasing our ability to operate machinery (including vehicles) safely. On the other hand, its beneficial effects include raising the good cholesterol (HDL), decreasing blood-clotting factors that can cause heart attacks, improving some individual social graces, as well as accentuating relaxation. Certainly, if a patient has a tendency to overdrink, a family history of alcoholism, or religious conflicts, he or she should avoid alcohol. Also, the detriments of operating heavy equipment or driving even after one drink more than offsets any benefit alcohol might provide.

Alcohol is a plant product, and therefore, a carbohydrate full of calories (seven per gram). Thus, if a person drinks, he or she must decrease overall food intake to avoid getting fat. Consumed in excess, alcohol can raise the blood triglycerides and place fat in the liver in some susceptible individuals.

Chronic excess alcohol consumption leads to many health problems, including elevated blood pressure, uric acid, and over a long period of time, tissue damage in the liver (cirrhosis), muscles, brain, and heart. Women, because of their metabolic differences, should generally drink half as much alcohol as men.

As mentioned before (see Page 170), wine, particularly the reds, is my recommendation because it contains a variety of antioxidants and is more beneficial than other types of alcoholic products. No more than six ounces should be drunk in a ninety-minute period, and only while eating, since food slows down the absorption of alcohol. Antioxidants like resveratol, which is most concentrated in muscatel and sangiovese, are produced by grapes to ward off infecting invaders to the fruit. In humans, resveratol has been shown to stimulate nerve cell connections and may be helpful in preventing Alzheimer's disease. Resveratol has been isolated and sold in capsules, and is also found in dark grape juice, although its concentration there is one-fifth of that in wine. Neither of these alcohol-free sources are as effective as red wine, however, because they do not contain alcohol itself as well as other micronutrients.

A major Harvard study conducted by Dr. Gary Curham showed that of 81,093 women ages forty to sixty-five, those who had a daily eight-ounce glass of wine reduced their risk of having kidney stones by 59 percent. The same amount of tea, regular, or decaffeinated coffee would reduce the risk by only 9 percent. Recently, beer has also been shown to prevent kidney stones, as well as osteoporosis. Scientists believe the hops in beer is the beneficial agent.

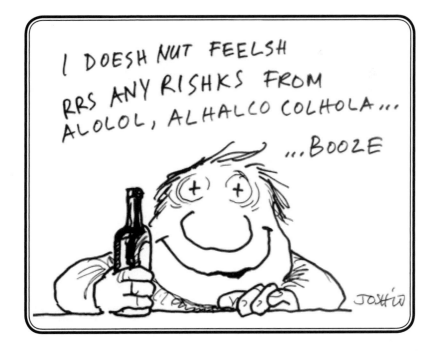

5

Forever Young

Death

You are going to die! We as humans will not win that war. However, armed with prudent and healthy living, combined with the facts we now know to be effective and what we surmise to be helpful in the future, we can win many battles and postpone the final encounter. This will enable us to have both quality and quantity of life—we will live both better and longer. In the year 2010, it is predicted that one of three babies born will become a centenarian. However, a pessimistic but scientifically researched statement appeared in *JAMA* saying that unless we change our paradigm of eating and working in the twenty-first century, the epidemic of obesity will prevent our children from living even as long as their parents.

As a physician, I have often wondered if we should consider aging to be a disease and treat it as such. Certainly both primary and secondary aging are under genetic control. There are well-described premature aging diseases such as progeria (the body of a twenty-year-old is functionally eighty) and Alzheimer's disease (the premature aging of the mind). On the other hand, the "Methuselah gene" was predicted in 1992, and we are still looking for it. This might be responsible for the cellular production of a powerful antioxidant, superoxide dismutase (SOD), by which one could stay physically young until age 120. The genetic aspect of aging is being worked out in the Human Genome Project, which has determined the site of each of the 3.2 billion genes. This is the code of all codes, *ours*. It has shown several of these genes, among them SIR1 and SIR2, promote longevity. Resveratol, the constituent in wine, turns on that gene, and that is one of the reasons many scientists claim that wine is so healthy in moderation. This substance can now be concentrated from other sources, and doses equivalent to drinking 100 gallons of wine a day can be consumed in just one capsule.

The human genome sequence will be the foundation of biology for decades and centuries to come. It is comparable to the periodic elemental table initiated over a century ago and was the basis for the discovery of almost a hundred new elements, including radioactive ones that led to nuclear energy production. Already, researchers are extracting DNA (genetic material) from blood, attaching fluorescent molecules, and sprinkling them on a special glass chip. This chip has its surface embedded with 5,000 known genes. A laser reads the fluorescence, which indicates which of the known genes on the chip are in the mystery sample from a patient.

The very expensive Afymax 5KR is available now for some genetic readouts, but in the future, more of this knowledge of gene expression will give us the power to re-engineer the human species and gradually improve quality of life by attacking both secondary (degenerative) diseases and primary aging (just getting old). The three-plus billion genes are on twenty-three paired chromosomes, which are labeled as chromosome 1, chromosome 2, and the two sex chromosomes identified as x and y.

Proteomics has emerged from genomics with the discovery that one gene can make at least ten different proteins. Many potential diseases will hence be cured epigenetically on a molecular level even before they arise. Pharmacogenetics, now practiced by many doctors, will indicate not just how an individual will metabolize a drug (fast or slow), but whether a given drug will work for an individual patient. This is frequently done for treatments with anticoagulents (Plavix, Coumadin), seizure meds (Dilantin), and antimetabolites (Imuran). This is also done in Tamoxifin for breast cancer. One also can prevent a gene from making a harmful protein such as the B-amyloid of Alzheimer's disease by injecting "antisense" molecules to foil the protein production. Although we cannot change our God-given genes, we can certainly now modify them, such as turning off or on the good and bad expressions of individual chromosomes. The use of Genelex, Athrotec, and Spectrocell in delineating the genetic CVP, APO-E is commonly used by modern doctors. Therefore, aging is a definite but not an immutable process of living.

On a cellular level, at birth, our cells are programmed to multiply only so many times before they individually die. This highly organized form of cell death, called apoptosis, is critical for both our health and our demise. When the process malfunctions too little, programmed cell death results in cancer or autoimmune diseases, while too much causes acceleration of the degenerative diseases. At the end of the process, suicide is committed by the cells; they chop themselves up into membrane-wrapped chunks. Cells compose tissues, which cumulatively make up our organs. And of course, we are made up of organs (heart, kidney, lungs, etc.). The natural decline of our cells (tissues and organs) is aging and adding an insult to injury with degenerative disease processes could result in a catastrophic event for that organ system, causing death of the human being.

We infrequently doubt our beliefs, but we too often believe our doubts. A recent survey by the Harvard School of Public Health shows that most of us have a pessimistic outlook about certain diseases. For example, women put their odds of developing breast cancer at 40 percent, whereas it is actually 10 percent. Men say that prostate cancer strikes down 30 percent of their fellow males, but the truth is only 10 percent of men get the disease. The probability of being seriously injured in an auto accident, people felt, was 50 percent, when it is actually 5 percent. Nearly everyone doubled their risk of stroke, heart attack, diabetes, or HIV from the true statistic. Life expectancy certainly has increased in the last century, but most of this is not due to breakthroughs in treating disease by our high tech methods, but to better obstetrical techniques, improvement in prenatal mortality, and control of infectious diseases in childhood through immunization. It is true that we have pushed the envelope a little and postponed death by expensive procedures such as organ transplants. Most of the prolongation of life in the near future will still be through preventive methods such as intervening early in our genetic environment, avoiding smoking, eating sensibly, eating gluten-free (for the 25 percent of our population that is intolerant), remaining physically active, and by keeping a "clean" house. The latter includes drinking clean water and PEP (see chart on opposite page).

As was mentioned above, our goal should be not just living longer, but living better. My patients often say to me that they don't want to live to be old with all the hardships it entails. But on the other hand, who wants to be old when one is still relatively young? I know people in their fifties who feel old and sick, and others in their eighties who are healthy and spry. It is not how old you are chronologically (your age), but how old you are physiologically (your internal functions) and physically (external appearance) that counts. Overall life expectancy in the United States reached a high of 77.9 in 2007, much lower than in fourteen other developed countries. It increased more for blacks than whites due to a "catch up" in the previously poor medical care African Americans received. The leading cause of death in people ages one to forty-four is injury; age forty-five to sixty-four it is cancer; and above sixty-five it is cardiovascular disease.

Put PEP* in Your Life

Here are some easy things anyone can do to improve their environment and therefore improve their health.

1. Take your shoes off when you come in the front door.
2. Move electric clocks and radios away from the bedside.
3. Use healthier cleaning materials.
4. Hang dry-cleaned clothes outside without plastic bag.
5. Change laundry soap and stop using dryer sheets loaded with chemicals.
6. Use white vinegar in last wash cycle to make clothes softer.
7. Never use chlorine bleach.
8. Open windows to let fresh air inside.
9. Eat more organic food.
10. Move keyboard farther away from your computer.
11. Keep children at least 10 feet away from the TV.
12. Clean out your refrigerator, and clean the drain pan to get rid of mold.
13. Buy a few plants good for the environment, such as a spider plant.
14. Use candles made of beeswax or vegetable oil.
15. No lead based wicks.
16. Check to make sure your dryer, is vented properly to the outside.
17. Cancel the pest control plan and use neutral agents like Borax.
18. Use stainless steel or glass cookware.
19. Buy a shower filter to absorb chlorine.
20. Use tobacco for pest control for plants.

* Personal Environmental Protection

We do have to get older, but we do not have to age as we get older. Genetically and even biblically speaking (see Genesis 6:3), we should live to be 120. To examine how to live longer, we need to look into why certain individuals such as Jean Calmet of France died at age 122 in 1997. This, then, is studying the oldest of the old such as the government-funded study currently being done in Baltimore. Dan Buettner's *Blue Zones* explains some of the mechanisms for some subpopulations to live to a ripe, old, healthy age. Medicine explains it nicely: degenerative diseases superimposed on primary aging. A machine, particularly a human one, will not last forever. We know that infection, trauma, heart disease, and cancer do cause our demise, but even if there were none of these, primary aging will eventually kill us. It is a fact of life that we will all die, hence the old adage, "The two basic truths in life are, we will pay taxes and we will die" (despite the new tax law that we will not have to pay as much tax when we die!). So, we will all die sometime. Hopefully, that time will be when we are close to our target of 120 years. The Telomere test will give a good idea of your forthcoming morbidity and mortality. We cannot change our genes, but we can certainly modify them by lifestyle change. This test can be done every six months (if you can afford it) to see if you are winning or losing your game of life.

In April 2010, the *New England Journal of Medicine* detailed the trajectories during the last five years of life: The categories include no disability, catastrophic, accelerated, progressive, and persistently severe. Most of those who died suddenly had no disability. Those who died from dementia had persistent severe disability. The degree of frailty increased dramatically from the sudden death to the lingering death. The study involved 754 community-dwelling older persons. The picture would be far different if drawn from nursing home or hospital populations, which have much more frailty. The costs associated with hospitalized persons during their last year of life may be equal to the total health care expenditure of all previous years.

A long life is not necessarily synonymous with a healthy one, but I want to discuss a long, healthy life as was the design of our Creator—followed by an immediate transfer to peace, oblivion, heaven, or whatever your belief system tells you follows this life. Whether the Big Bang Theorym evolution or God created the earth and all within it, is a moot point with regard to our health. Whether we are here by chance, luck, or as I feel, by the hand of God, makes little difference to healthy living. The fact is, we are here, and we should and can live life to its fullest and at its best. Many of us feel that we don't mind death as much as we mind dying! Or, as the late George Burns said, "I don't want to be there when it happens." Therefore, it is not about prolonging death with all its suffering, but prolonging life and all the goodness it entails; and then that sudden and perhaps a beautiful transition to the hereafter. At the end, we will simply go to sleep, then "wake up dead." In the future, I believe conscious sedation until death at the end of life will be the norm rather than the exception.

THE IMPACT OF DISEASE

Disease certainly will change the ideal life curve (see Figure IV-1). Some diseases are promptly announced at the beginning of the process, such as an overwhelming infection like pneumonia. But others are very subtle like atherosclerosis, and it is years or even decades before they become noisy and recognized. Defeating the disease process at its inception, or better yet, before it is introduced into our tissues, such as in embryos or at birth, should be medicine's goal. This could be better accomplished through genetic testing of cord blood at birth rather than by family history. Then, hopefully, we can take measures to reverse (through gene therapy), to prevent, or to greatly retard the course of disease. In describing life, we need to consider both morbidity and vitality, which are inversely related. One hundred percent vitality has no morbidity, and conversely, there is no vitality in death, which is 100 percent morbid. Figure V-2 may help to detail this better. An earlier identification and a therapeutic intervention (see Figure V-3) will decrease morbidity and delay mortality.

It is far better if a disease is detected and stopped, allowing the person to live a full life and die at age 110. But this is not what we have in medical practice today. A degenerative disease process such as atherosclerosis (see Figure V-2) may have its onset at age twenty and slowly progress—because of genetic or environmental reasons such as smoking or an unhealthy diet—to age fifty. With a change of diet or lifestyle,

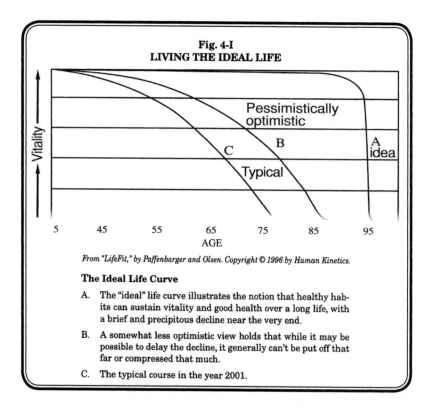

Fig. 4-I
LIVING THE IDEAL LIFE

From "LifeFit," by Paffenbarger and Olsen. Copyright © 1996 by Human Kinetics.

The Ideal Life Curve

A. The "ideal" life curve illustrates the notion that healthy habits can sustain vitality and good health over a long life, with a brief and precipitous decline near the very end.

B. A somewhat less optimistic view holds that while it may be possible to delay the decline, it generally can't be put off that far or compressed that much.

C. The typical course in the year 2001.

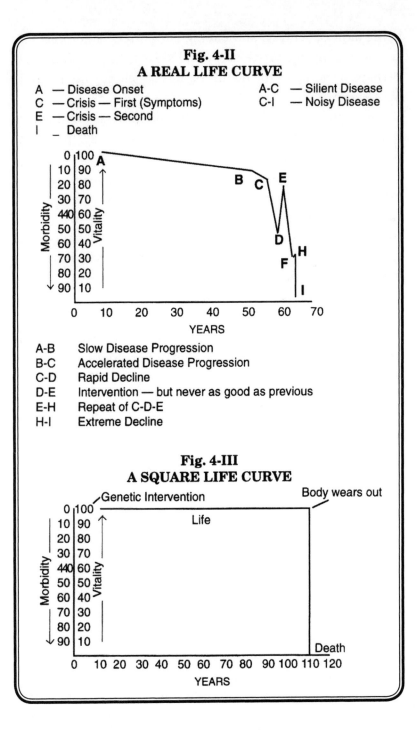

Fig. 4-II
A REAL LIFE CURVE

A — Disease Onset   A-C — Silient Disease
C — Crisis — First (Symptoms)   C-I — Noisy Disease
E — Crisis — Second
I _ Death

A-B   Slow Disease Progression
B-C   Accelerated Disease Progression
C-D   Rapid Decline
D-E   Intervention — but never as good as previous
E-H   Repeat of C-D-E
H-I   Extreme Decline

Fig. 4-III
A SQUARE LIFE CURVE

being more sedentary, and having more stress, atherosclerosis accelerates. By age fifty-eight, the disease is finally diagnosed, perhaps by going to the doctor because of chest pain and high cholesterol.

The atherosclerosis process still progresses, but medical intervention can help some and there may be some improvement. Then comes the "big one"—a heart attack at age sixty, which markedly alters one's health. The person survives, but now has congestive heart failure. He is hospitalized, but survives. However, he is never as well as he was before. The survival is only temporary, and within six months of a miserable existence in a nursing home, he dies. Again, returning to Figure V-3, with an earlier diagnosis, we can nip the disease in the bud and compact the downward spiral to a very short time before death.

It is that person's last small fraction of life that costs not only an inordinate amount of health care dollars, but for that poor individual an unbearable amount of misery. The patient, as well as the immediate family, indeed suffers. These misfortunes then do not prolong life, but only prolong the unhappy ending to what otherwise might be a full and rewarding life.

Presently, as we get older, we have more and more illnesses, which leave us more and more feeble, and hence we have a lingering death. We have all heard the expression that a patient looks like "death warmed over." The patient looks old, feels old, and indeed *is* chronologically old. The gradual descent into old age, older age, and then death is what is happening to most of us today, The ideal would be to be healthy until the last day or two of our existence and then die, or better yet, go to sleep one night and "wake up dead." Disability and functional impairment will then be compressed to a very brief time after an extremely lengthy period of health and vigor. In the *New England Journal of Medicine,* Dr. Anthony Vita examined data from the 1941 alumni of the University of Pennsylvania born between 1913 and 1925. The relationship to modifiable factors of smoking, body mass index, and exercise patterns indicated that better health habits not only increased survival, but more importantly, postponed and compressed disability to a shorter time at life's end. The time to be concerned about when and how we die is now while there is still time to do something about it.

A living will and a durable power of attorney are a must. This obligation is given to a friend, spouse, or adult child who not only knows you well, but who will fight for your right to die in the manner you choose. Some people want to live no matter the conditions, while others, if facing prolonged pain and suffering with no hope of recovery, choose to go quickly. Life support should not be initiated, and the phrase "Do Not Resuscitate" should be boldly recorded on your hospital chart.

If there is pain, conscious sedation should be initiated with drugs such as IV Propofol until the final time. In the future, I suspect society will become more accepting of euthanasia for those who choose it.

THE BIOLOGY OF AGING

Aging can be divided into a primary and secondary condition. Primary aging at the cellular level can be defined as a progressive deterioration of structure and function that occurs over time. Secondary aging is the superimposition of degenerative processes that progress with time. These include such entities as atherosclerosis, osteoarthritis, Alzheimer's disease, and other diseases, and all the handicaps that occur with them. Healthy or successful aging is the delaying of the cellular deterioration and the prevention of degradation for as long as possible. Shortly we will discuss the theories of aging, but restricting food intake and increasing exercise and hormone replacement have definitely been proven in the medical literature to retard primary aging in humans. The use of bioidentical hormones such as estrogen, progesterone, testosterone, human growth hormone, and thyroid hormones will greatly enhance the quality and quantity of our lives.

We all live to die, but some of us are dying to live. The final years of life will be far better if one continues to be enthusiastic, which also will help ensure longevity. It is contentment, complacency, and satisfaction, not excitement and exhilaration, that is important for lengthening our pleasurable lifespan. People age at different rates, and even within a given individual certain organ systems exhibit varying speeds of decline. Aging occurs throughout our body: the heart rate and force of contraction decrease, blood vessel diameter decreases, muscles lose mass, bones develop osteoporosis, lung capacity diminishes, skin loses collagen, hormonal production changes dramatically, and there are significant alterations in sensory functions. Some researchers refer to the pause of an organ system, such as menopause, as a sudden decline in the ovaries of a woman as a reflection of aging. The earlier the identification of the multiple pauses that comprise primary aging, the earlier and simpler the intervention will be and the more successful the outcomes.

The Aging of Our Body Parts

Brain

Some scientists believe aging begins in the brain with "electropause," a change in the P300, the positive brain wave, at 500 ohms. The loss of amplitude and/or voltage results in delays of neurotransmission in the cortex, with implications for every body organ and system.

Over time, the brain loses some neurons and others become damaged. The brain adapts to these changes, however, by increasing the number of synapses and by regenerating dendrites and axons. However, there is a toll with decreased memory and reaction time as the brain electrically and structurally ages.

Proper nourishment of our brain over time keeps our brain more dynamic (neuroplasticity) and younger than our given years. Omega 3s, coconut oil, DMAE, vinpocetine, procaine (part of the Gerivital potion), ginseng, ginko biloba, pregnenolone, phosphatidylserine, vincopocetine glutathione, piracetam, melatonin, huperzine A, and numerous antioxidants can help. Exercise and a good diet (especially one without gluten and preservatives, full of micronutrients served in a safe dish) will help grow brain cells, even in a centenarian. Stress, general anesthesia, head trauma, infections, drugs, depression, alcohol in excess, a sedentary lifestyle, lack of intellectual stimulation, decreased social contact, exposure to toxic environments (physical, such as radiation and pollutants, and psychological, such as strife and unforgiveness), and cardiovascular disease also contribute to a more rapid decline in brain function. Using all parts of our brain retards senility. Crossword puzzles, reading, and writing upside down can be helpful. The use of the non-dominant side such as writing with the left hand or sighting with the left eye (if right-handed) "grows" neurons and synapses. Of course, learning a new discipline or even dancing are excellent ways to prevent brain deterioration. Prevention of medical diseases and staying away from doctors with knives (unless it is essential for survival) will help brain function. Many drugs, such as statins, anticholenergics (to help control the bladder), and psychotropics, can add to brain deterioration.

Research has shattered the idea that we are born with all the brain cells (neurons) that we were ever going to have. The human brain has been coaxed into growing new nerve cells by a process called neurogenesis. Several mediators include Nrf-2 and brain-derived neurotropic factor (BDNF), which enhances neurogenesis. Every time a muscle contracts, it emits a special chemical that crosses the blood-brain barrier and stimulates BDNF and a host of neurotransmitters (chemicals that allow one nerve cell to talk to another). BDNF encourages the neurons to start sprouting, joining, and communicating with other nerve cells.

In addition to BDNF, resistance exercise allows the heart to pump more blood into the brain, resulting in more oxygenation, nourishment, and growth of new blood vessels. In the *Proceedings of the National Academy of Sciences*, Scott Small, a Columbia University neurologist, showed that BDNF increases the number of neurons, particularly in the hippocampus, which controls learning and memory, as well as the frontal lobes, the seat of executive function. The hippocampus helps the brain match names with faces, an ability that tends to decrease as we age. Executive function involves higher thought, which entails decision-making, planning, and multitasking. Dr. Kristine Byaffe, of the University of California in San Francisco, found in autopsies that athletes had more astrocytes (cells that support the neurons) and enhanced neurotransmitters (norepinephrine, serotonin, and dopamine).

New brain cells with these neurotransmitters, as well as a person's IQ, increase almost immediately after exercise. Furthermore, other studies show that people who exercise at least three times a week have a lower incidence of Alzheimer's, and those who do have Alzheimer's disease show less degeneration of brain function if they continue to exercise.

In addition to increased brain power, exercise creates a marked reduction of other degenerative diseases (coronary artery disease, stroke, diabetes, and cancer). Carole Lewis co-authored the book *Age-Defying Fitness*, which revealed that aerobic exercise (running, bicycling), anaerobic exercise (lifting weights and use of machines), and balancing exercises (using the Big Ball and the Bosu balance trainer), all seem to benefit brain function. EWOT (Exercise with Oxygen Therapy) boosts brain power even more. Exercise for the brain is important for youngsters, more so for adults, and essential for seniors. So as your body goes, your brain will follow.

Eyes

Essential for good sight is early detection of glaucoma, prevention and treatment of macular degeneration, cataract interception, and control of blood sugar in diabetes. Both age-related macular degeneration and cataracts may be prevented by antioxidants. The former demands early and intensive treatment, whereas the latter can continue until vision reaches a critical point, requiring surgery. Since we are as young as we look and feel, having good eyesight, particularly without glasses, is valuable in staying younger longer.

Your grandmother may have been correct that highly colored vegetables are good for your eyesight, but reading in low light and straining to read will not adversely affect vision. However, vision problems can make it difficult to read in low light.

Refractive Correcting Procedure

All refractive corneal surgery reshapes the cornea to redirect light rays so that they focus on the retina. In myopia (nearsightedness), rays converge in front of the retina; surgical flattening of the cornea focuses the rays farther back. In hyperopia (farsightedness), light rays strike the retina before they can focus; steepening the cornea makes the rays converge closer to the retina. In astigmatism, the cornea is not spherical because one meridian is steeper or flatter than the others; flattening a steep meridian or steepening a flat meridian tends to bring the light rays in focus nearer to the retina. The poor focusing of an image does cause blurring of our vision, as do other eye diseases. Glasses can correct 95 percent of refractive problems, plus there are surgical corrective measures.

GLAUCOMA

The symptoms of glaucoma are visual loss and blurred vision. Glaucoma is a partial loss of one's view caused by increased pressure in the eye fluid that damages the optic nerve. It affects one million Americans aged sixty-five and older, and it is the leading cause of blindness among African Americans.

Eight out of ten glaucoma cases are the open angle type and account for 10 percent of cases of legal blindness in the United States. Risk factors include family history, increased age, extreme nearsightedness, hypertension, diabetes, and long-term corticosteroid therapy. The disease develops more frequently and earlier among African Americans, and may be detected as early as age forty. Patients often remain asymptomatic until the disease has progressed significantly. The American Academy of Ophthalmology recommends that people older than forty-five undergo comprehensive eye examinations every two years, and every year if they have risk factors for glaucoma. Closed angle glaucoma develops in 20 percent of cases and is more symptomatic and dangerous. Several types of medications and/or surgery may reduce intraocular pressure.

CATARACT

The symptoms of cataract are blurred vision, glare, and double vision. Opacitites in the lens of the eye, or cataracts, affect fewer than 5 percent of persons under sixty-five but almost half of Americans aged seventy-five and older. The *Archives of Ophthalmology* reported people taking vitamins C and E for greater than ten years had a 60 percent reduced risk of cataracts.[5] The most common cause of blindness worldwide, cataracts are a less important cause of vision impairment in the United States because of the availability and efficacy of outpatient cataract surgery. More than 1.5 million such procedures are performed each year, and 90 percent of treated patients enjoy a significant visual improvement, with a 1 percent complication rate. These are several types of procedures. Choose an ophthalmologist who has done hundreds of them and has a good reputation.

DIABETIC AND METABOLIC SYNDROME EYE DISEASE (RETINOPATHY)

The symptoms are blurred vision, floaters, visual field loss, and poor right vision. Diabetic retinopathy affects many middle-aged and older Americans who are at risk of Type 2 diabetes. Diabetic retinopathy may escape detection for some time. Ten to 20 percent of people diagnosed with Type 2 diabetes concurrently have retinopathy. Patients who complain of blurry vision or distorted central vision may have "background," or nonproliferative diabetic retinopathy, which is caused by hemorrhages or fluid collection. Proliferative diabetic retinopathy involves the growth of new, abnormal blood vessels in the retina that leak, impair vision, and may cause retinal detachment. Various surgical approaches and laser treatment are effective in both forms of diabetic retinopathy. In people with diabetes, good blood sugar control is believed to prevent or delay the onset of diabetic retinopathy and slow its progression once it has occurred.

MACULAR DEGENERATION

Macular degeneration affects more than 15 million people in the United States. The macula is a small area in the retina that is needed for central vision. It provides the focus used to perform fine work, such as reading and sewing. Higher risk is noted in smokers, those who have been overexposed to sunlight, women, and people with lighter-colored (blue, green, and hazel) eyes. Cataracts of varying degree frequently accompany macular degeneration. There are two types; the wet, which occurs in 10 percent of the people with macular degeneration, and the dry, which is noted in the remaining 90 percent. The wet type is much more aggressive and gets its

DO YOU HAVE MACULAR DEGENERATION?

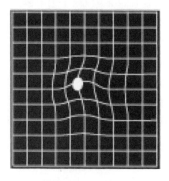

Abnormal

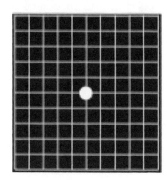

Normal

Testing your vision with the Amsler Grid:

You can check your vision daily by using an Amsler grid like the one pictured above on the right. You may find changes in your vision that you wouldn't notice otherwise. Xeroxing or cutting the grid and putting it on the front of your refrigerator is a good way to remember to look at it each day, or just open to this page. There is both a wet (more rapid and severe) and a dry (more common) type.

To use the grid:

1. Wear your reading glasses and hold this grid at 12-15 inches in good light.
2. Cover one eye.
3. Look directly at the center dot with the uncovered eye.
4. While looking directly at the center dot, note whether all lines of the grid are straight or if any areas are distorted, blurred or dark as the one on the left.
5. Repeat this procedure with the other eye.
6. If any area of the grid looks wavy, blurred or dark, such as on the left, contact your ophthalmologist immediately.

name from the bleeding capillaries within the macula. The dry type (also called age-related), which usually progresses over years or decades, is caused by deterioration of the macular cells. These are pigmented structures, and blue light hastens their dysfunction, and later destruction.

Antioxidants, vitamins, zeaxanthin, lutein, Omega 3 fish oils, and zinc retard and/or prevent dry macular degeneration. For the wet variety, laser has been used to stop the capillary bleeding, although it also destroys some of the good capillaries and other cells. An old technique has been refined for the treatment of the wet disease. The drug is called verteporfin (Visudyne). The ophthalmologist targets the vessel with a low-power laser that "turns on" the drug, which causes micro blood clots in the small vessels and hence, seals them off. This treatment is effective in 30 percent of those with wet macular degeneration. Intravenous injections of EDTA (Chelation) have been shown to be effective in both dry and wet macular degeneration, as well as for cataracts. See Figure V-5 to determine if you have macular degeneration. Blurred vision, image distortion, and holes in the visual field are symptoms of macular degeneration. Using the grid frequently will allow you to determine if you have this disease and allow you to seek immediate ophthalmologic care.

HEART

The heart grows slightly larger with age. Maximal oxygen consumption during exercise declines in men by about 10 percent and in women by about 7.5 percent with each decade of adult life. Cardiac output stays nearly the same, however, because the heart actually pumps more efficiently. Exercise, both aerobic and resistance, will keep the heart muscle stronger longer. Nutrients such as MCT (medium chain triglycerides, or coconut oil), d-ribose, and l-carnitine will make the heart muscle work better. Magnesium and selenium will not only enhance the heart effort, but also maintain its electrical action (arrhythmia prevention). Herbs such as hawthorne berry improve the heart contraction and its rhythm. Coenzyme Q10, which is naturally depleted in the elderly and earlier with statin therapy, increases heart contraction. The no-longer-in-fashion herb digitalis still should be considered in refractory heart failure, but it is prescriptive and most doctors don't know how to give it. Coronary artery disease is the most prevalent type of heart problem, but in most cases it can be prevented by diet and exercise.

Lungs

Maximum breathing capacity may decline by about 40 percent between the ages of twenty and eighty years. Exercise, particularly "cardio," with bursts of extreme activity (see page 77) can improve lung capacity. Staying away from airborne pollution from autos (particularly diesel), secondhand cigarette smoke, indoor fireplaces, and industrial fumes keep the respiratory system healthier. Improving the immune system and taking annual flu shots go a long way to prevent pulmonary problems later in life.

Blood Vessels

The veins age more slowly than the arteries. They become baggy and dilated, particularly in the legs. The valves that control the flow of blood to the heart become dilated and incompetent with subsequent further dilation of the vein and an increase of venous pressure (varicose veins). Sometimes they leak red blood cells, causing discoloration of the adjacent skin. Also, fluid leaks out, resulting in swelling or edema of the adjacent tissue. Because of hypercoagulation, blood clots can form within. If there is inflammation in the vessel it is called thrombophlebitis and tends to be more painful, but it does not migrate through the heart to the lungs (pulmonary embolus) as does the noninflamed (venous thrombosis). If there is no surrounding inflammation (phlebothrombosis), the clot does not adhere to the wall and is much more dangerous because it can embolise to the lung.

The arteries are the vessels that carry the oxygenated blood from the heart to the tissues. Arterial walls thicken as systolic blood pressure increases 20 to 25 percent between ages twenty and seventy-five years. This hardening of the artery causes even less elasticity, and the pressure within goes even higher, with more damage. This vicious negative cycle continues until either a catastrophe occurs or something reverses the process. The consequences are arteriosclerosis (hardening), atherosclerosis (soft cholesterol plaque), a thrombosis (clot) develops on top of the plaque, causing obstruction of the vessel or, in rare cases, an aneurysm—rupture of the artery itself!

HYPERTENSION

Much debate exits in the world of hypertension. However, there are some facts that are incontrovertible. There is no doubt that the older the person, the higher the blood pressure. The longer and the higher the blood pressure, the more damage to the blood vessels, and hence the organs of the body. Because our cardiovascular system takes the brunt of the injury, it comes as no surprise that heart attacks and strokes occur because of high blood pressure. Not so well known is that the kidneys suffer even earlier. This is a subtle problem, and unless simple renal functions are tested, the patient and doctor will not know about it. The Plac2 test best describes how and when an event will happen. But kidney damage provokes accelerated damage to circulation. Since the inside lining of the blood vessels (endothelium) takes a beating, these delicate cells "protect" themselves by getting harder and thicker, leading to more atherosclerosis. Lifestyle, genetics, and the stressors in our lives will determine our blood pressure. The "rule of forties" is: Forty percent of our population over forty has elevated blood pressure, but only 40 percent know it. Of those who have it, 40 percent are treated, but only 40 percent are done so adequately!

The systolic (digits on the top) of the two numbers should be 115. But the bottom of the fraction, or the diastolic, is unsettled. In the past doctors recommended that it be well under 90. But now many physicians feel that the lower the diastolic, the worse the outlook for the patient. The difference between the two is the pulse pressure, the systolic minus the diastolic. The higher this number, the worse it is for the individual. When the figure is greater than 50, concern begins. Therefore, the person whose blood pressure is 130/60 is in worse cardiac condition than the one who has a blood pressure of 130/70. So I do not even note the diastolic number in most cases. Suffice it to say, if we keep the systolic number less than 125, the diastolic is usually fine. Of course, if the systolic drops from a previous "normal" to less than 115, then something unhealthy is happening.

Blood pressure has a normal daily variation. It is usually higher in the morning and lower in the evening. "White Coat Hypertension" (a person's blood pressure rising in the doctor's office) does occur, and it is not to be taken lightly. Those who have this do not live as long as those whose blood pressure does not rise in the doctor's office. And if the blood pressure is transiently elevated higher than 200, attention should be paid immediately. An older set of pipes (blood vessels) is more likely to break at peak pressure rather than at a lower one. So the sooner the blood pressure is normalized, the better.

There are several methods to obtain a person's blood pressure. The gold standard is the sphygmomanometer, but the airoid gauge and electronic cuffs work equally well. The larger the circumference of the arm, the wider the cuff diameter needed and vice versa. If a cuff is too narrow, there will be a false elevation of the reading. The person should be sitting comfortably for five minutes, with the arm resting on a surface at heart level before the blood pressure is taken. Wrist cuffs and finger devices are not as accurate. An even better evaluation of the artery and its pressure is with a plethymagraph, which can be done anywhere from the upper arm to the finger.

THE PHYSIOLOGY/PATHOLOGY OF HYPERTENSION

The blood needs pressure in order to push it throughout the body. This comes from the active kinetic force of the heart and the passive potential power of the elastic arteries, especially the big ones such as the aorta and its subsequent first branches— brachial and femoral. The former is responsible for the systolic and the latter for the diastolic blood pressure. Some scientists think that there is no such thing as blood pressure. Rather, they believe it is an epiphenomenon, a reflection of the health of the blood vessel and specifically the inside lining, the endothelium. When the endothelial cells become stressed and dysfunctional, they communicate with the overlying smooth muscle and they contract, making the artery smaller and thus putting more force on the arterial wall. We medically make these constricted vessels healthier by using smooth muscle relaxants (ARBs, calcium blockers, and ace inhibitors). This releases the tense muscles, and the internal force diminishes.

If there is an increase of sympathetic stimulation, the heart beats stronger and the blood pressure goes up. Doctors use drugs that decrease the sympathetic tone (beta blockers). The kidney is intimately involved in vasomotor control, in that it produces a hormone (rennin) that causes smooth muscle contraction. Also, the less blood that goes to the kidney, because of hypertensive damage to the blood vessels that supply it, the more rennin is produced and the more contraction of the arterial muscle, which still further reduces the renal blood flow, and the pressure goes even higher. It becomes a vicious cycle. There are groups of drugs that decrease rennin both directly and indirectly (ARBS [Diovan], ACES [Vasotec], DRIS [Tekturna]). Another way high blood pressure is produced is through salt and water in extreme excess; doctors use diuretics for these cases.

Causes of Hypertension

Atherosclerosis compromises the endothelial cells, causing the blood vessel to actively narrow and the pressure to go up. This process also occurs in the renal arteries, and the hormone rennin comes pouring out. Through several pathways, the arteries contract even more. In other cases excess fluid and salt accumulate within the body, which results in more water in the artery and hence the blood pressure goes up. The adrenal gland makes another hormone, aldosterone. If there is too much "aldo" from either a benign tumor or an enlargement of this portion of the gland, then the blood pressure elevates. Aldo also lowers one's potassium, and if a diuretic is given to the patient to treat the blood pressure, it could cause a very low potassium content—enough to cause the heart to become irritable and in extreme cases to even stop!

Non-Drug Treatment

The desire of many people is to not take medications unless nothing else works. I therefore recommend lifestyle changes first. Exercise with weight loss is a given, and 60 percent of folks will normalize their blood pressure if they will do it, though this is difficult. Cutting down on salt with the use of over-the-counter potassium and magnesium, really helps. For the former, I recommend the use of NoSalt or NuSalt, which can be obtained at the grocery store. Even if one never uses salt I tell them to use these products. A half teaspoon a day is my advice, so use this "salt shaker" heavily, even in cooking. At first it may seem bitter, but in two weeks it will taste like regular salt, and if you were to use real salt, then it would seem way too salty. Your taste buds will adjust. For magnesium, I recommend a mag chelate. A chelate is an organic salt such as citrate, aspartate, glycinate, etc. Calm is a mag citrate powder, available at health food stores. Two teaspoons a day should do good things for your blood pressure (and also your nerves, heart, migraines, and muscle cramps). It comes in several flavors. I like lemon, and I put it in my smoothies. Dark chocolate is another natural product. However, most chocolates have a fair amount of sugar and fats, therefore baking chocolate or unsweetened cocoa is recommended. They can be put in coffee or used to make fudge with the biologic sugar substitute xylitol. The flesh of sardines contains a natural peptide similar to a safe and effective blood pressure medication. Eight stalks of celery, three cups hibiscus tea, 400 mg of alpha lipoic acid, CoQ10, and 3,000 mg of Omega 3s are other natural ways to decrease blood pressure.

BREATHING EXERCISES

Breathing exercises also lower blood pressure. An FDA-approved device called a respirate is on the market (see www.respirate.com), costing about $300. It works well in lowering blood pressure by tracking the respiratory rate. With music, the machine instructs the listener to breathe slowly in and out in harmony with the music ascending and descending. This decreases the sympathetic nervous activity, which enhances relaxation and consequently lowers blood pressure. With this procedure, the exhalation takes at least 50 percent more time than the inhalation. A less expensive method, without using any fancy equipment, is a technique called high five. With this method, one inhales through the nose for a count of five, holds the breath for a count of five, then exhales the air through the nose for a count of five. When exhaling, the tip of the tongue should be touching the roof of the mouth, immediately in back of the front teeth. This is a yoga position that enhances relaxation. I do this five times a day: first thing in the morning before even getting out of bed, last thing at night after I say my prayers, and three times a day when I think about it. If you do this four times a day you will still be doing well. If you can't remember to do them, do it once before each meal. It will also relax you for the forthcoming meal, which will enhance digestion.

Medicines for Blood Pressure

There are classes of drugs, and each class may have six to eight individual preparations. Also, there are various combinations of these classes. To add to the confusion, each drug has a generic and several brand names for the same medication. Of the over 400 antihypertensives available, one gets "the most bang for the buck" with the generic Lisinopril (2.5 to 40 mg daily). The most potent and also inexpensive is the generic Minoxidil (2.5 to 100 mg daily). With the latter, diuretics and beta-blockers are prescribed conjointly to limit the side effects of fluid retention and increased heart rate with high doses of this medication.

Treatment

In salt-sensitive individuals, primarily African Americans, diuretics may be needed. But many doctors use diuretics indiscriminately. It is true that some studies show that they are effective and cheap. The most common one used is hydrochlorithiazide, but I do not use it because it promotes loss of both potassium and magnesium and raises blood sugar and uric acid, which can create more heart problems. It is not enough just to treat the blood pressure, but it must be treated to a goal of less than 125. The scientific literature reveals that for every point above 115, there is a small decrease in life expectancy. It may be no big deal if a blood pressure is fifteen points above ideal, or that one dies two years sooner, but the greater problem would be to have a disability! Not only could there be heart failure in the future, but a heart attack, and—a fate worse than death—a stroke! Therefore, a good physician would endeavor to use an inexpensive drug with minimum side effects to get that patient to their ideal blood pressure, which is as close to 115 as possible without the individual becoming extremely lightheaded upon standing. When prescribing, we try not to push the dose of any one drug too high to avoid toxicity, and rather than change completely to another class of drug, new meds are added. Rarely can this be done with just one drug; frequently two or three medications must be given. In the past, there were single short-acting meds, so many pills several times a day were needed. Now there are various combinations of two and even three long-acting drugs in several doses available for convenience, so two pills instead of nine are taken daily.

PANCREAS

The pancreas has two functions: endocrine (hormone) and exocrine (enzymes). Regarding the hormone insulin, if we are lucky enough to be born with the right genetics, and had minimal or no cow's milk, gluten, or certain viral infections in our early childhood, Type 1 diabetes will not be in our future. However, the survival gene, which is survival of the fattest not the fittest, can cause a premature pancreatic exhaustion and Type 1 diabetes. The insulin receptors on our muscle, liver, and fat cells become resistant to the usual levels of insulin, and as more of this pours out of the pancreas, it fatigues and the sugar starts to rise. The already stressed pancreas becomes overworked; some cellular elements become weary and do not produce enough insulin for the already damaged tissue receptors.

The pancreatic enzymes needed for the digestion of food also become exhausted, and less of this potential life force is excreted when we eat. So, despite eating a healthy diet, the micro- and macronutrients are not being assimilated. Some practitioners feel that if extra food enzymes are ingested with and between meals, we will not dissipate these life-giving chemicals.

As we age, other problems can also injure this organ. Inflammation (pancreatitis), malignancy, obstruction from a gallstone, and trauma are the most common.

Urinary System

The kidneys gradually become less efficient at extracting waste from the blood. Bladder capacity declines. Urinary incontinence, which may occur after tissues atrophy, can often be managed through exercise, hormones, and behavioral techniques. The prostate enlarges, but can be treated with prescriptive or herbal preparations (saw palmetto, African pyregeum, pumpkin seed, etc.). The most common cause of kidney failure is age. Cardiovascular disease exacerbates the problem, and moderate kidney failure accelerates cardiovascular disease. Drugs, poisons, contrast studies (CT scans—see page 44), infections, and trauma also take their toll. In a healthy body, kidney function is measured by the creatine clearance test. Normal is 100 when young but decreases 10 percent a decade after age forty. When the value declines to 20, this is enough failure to warrant a transplant if we are lucky enough, or dialysis if not.

Body Fat

The body does not lose fat with age but redistributes it from just under the skin to deeper parts of the body. Women are more likely to store it in the hips and thighs, while men store it in the abdominal area. The real problem, however, is with decreasing thermogenesis and hormones as we age. The brown fat in the paravertebra area declines in function. The Lord, in all His wisdom, intelligently designed us so as we became older and less able to labor, eat, and digest, our bodies would become more efficient with our food and we would not starve. Unfortunately, in the land of plenty and little physical work, we accumulate too much fat. In the past, fat was stored up for times of famine and hard work. Now it is a liability, causing insulin intolerance and the release of destructive chemicals (cytochymes).

MUSCLES

Without exercise, estimated muscle mass declines 22 percent for women and 23 percent for men between the ages of thirty and seventy. Hand grip strength decreases 45 percent by age seventy-five. Exercise, especially resistance training, can help prevent much of this loss.

Sarcopenia (not enough muscle) and osteopenia (not enough bone) go hand in hand in the same person. Both decrease the quantity and, more importantly, the quality of life. Our ability to perform the most basic tasks that we need to stay independent falls off drastically as we lose our muscle mass. The risk of falling and injury increases, and our metabolic reserves decrease. Our muscles are the reservoir for needed protein when a medical illness befalls us. Muscle mass naturally falls off some in our forties, but we lose a great deal in our seventies. The main causes are less exercise and a lack of essential foods and hormones.

Aerobics such as jogging and biking are helpful, but not nearly as good as resistance exercises (weights, machines). Protein from whey (a milk fraction) is best to build up muscles. It has almost all the essential amino acids the body needs and none of the bad effects of milk from casein, lactose, and homogenized fat. Consuming the wrong protein (soy, cereal, and animal) leads to a mild acidosis, which causes a decrease of bone and muscle.

The anabolic hormones (DHEA, testosterone) naturally

decrease as we age. When measured, the normal range is far from ideal. For example, in most labs, testosterone levels are 200 to 1,200, but this is from ages nine to ninety-nine. For a young, healthy man, it is closer to 1,200. The so-called normal DHEA levels do not reflect the ideal in a human at peak health. Therefore, replacement of these hormones, particularly testosterone, prevents muscle and bone wasting, as well as having a generalized anti-aging effect.

Other ways to improve muscle mass include taking potassium bicarbonate to buffer acidosis; creatinine, the main protein of muscle; vitamin D for better neuromuscular coordination; and to a lesser extent, glutamine, carnitine, d-ribose, coconut oil, cinnamon, and Omega 3s. We should do all we can to maintain our muscles all our lives, rather than wait until we become a feeble invalid and it's too late. Then our life is terrible and for all intents and purposes, over. If you are reading this, it is not too late. Muscle is the protein storage we use for that unfortunate time when we are stressed by disease and cannot consume enough protein for sustenance. Work on your muscle conditioning now to prevent a miserable and early ending to your life.

EARS

More than 36 million Americans have some degree of hearing loss currently, but by the year 2030 it will be 80 million! Commonly, loud noises cause deafness; rarely it is congenital (birth defect) or acquired (infection of the brain or ears). In the past, the Woodstock Generation suffered hearing loss from loud noises caused by listening to rock concerts. Now we have the iPod generation, and the problem is still amplified music. With the popular digital audio players, which have exceptional clarity, listeners turn up the volume and send the loud sounds directly down the ear canal. The older analogue audio speakers had some distortion, which served as a natural volume governor, in that the louder the noise, the less clear it became. Hence, the listener would intentionally keep the volume less.

Regular use of aspirin, acetaminophen, and non-steroidal anti-inflammatory drugs, the most commonly used drugs in the United States, can increase the risk of hearing loss. The increased risk of hearing loss associated with regular analgesic use is greater among young men, particularly under the age of sixty.

Low dose aspirin (365 mg or less) has actually been shown to *protect* against hearing loss. Altering the Aldactone/aldosterone ratio will improve hearing.

In this noisy world, televisions are bigger and louder; movie theaters are much louder than decades ago; concerts are still available; and in the big cities, road construction, sirens, and traffic turn up the decibels. The intensity and duration of the noise causes the sensitive hearing hairs in the inner ear to be damaged. At 85 decibels for one hour (a lawn mower motor), damage can occur. Chainsaws are 100, and snowmobiles are 120 decibels. Rock concerts and digital ear devices can exceed 140 decibels. Genetically speaking, some people are more likely to have hearing loss, such as fair-skinned, male Caucasians compared to African Americans. The older we are, the more accumulation of toxic noises we receive. The ears were designed to pick up the faintest sounds of predators stalking our ancient ancestors, such as the snap of a twig in the forest, or the rustle of the grass on the Savannah, and not the crash and racket of modern life (motorcycles, subways, and car alarms).

Simple earplugs are recommended for most, but in a very noisy environment such as working outside an airport, hearing abatement devices are mandatory. Loss initially occurs in the high pitch range, but as time goes on, the middle frequencies, such as are made by the human voice, are lost. Hearing aids are amplifiers that are placed in the ear. The analogue device hearing aids cost from $300 to top-of-the-line digital technology for $3,000 plus. The latter has directional and high-definition hearing with two "microphones" and an algorithm to enhance the sound coming from the front of the person talking, while tuning down those from behind. Unfortunately, these are not paid for by insurance, they are minimally uncomfortable, and people, particularly men, do not want to wear these devices because it reveals them to be less than perfect. The use of an in-ear invisible device, such as the Lyric, makes life so much more pleasant and communication far better.

Tinnitus

Tinnitus, which occurs in 12 percent of the population, is the awareness of a sound that does not originate from an external source.

The term *tinnitus* is derived from Latin, meaning "to ring like a bell," although sufferers report hearing a variety of sounds from buzzing, humming, clanging to even roaring. There is no external source for these sounds since it is related to the auditory nerve transmitting impulses to the brain, which perceives them as this type of noise. Some patients take these symptoms without concern while in others it disrupts work and sleep.

There are two main types of tinnitus, subjective and objective. The much more common is the subjective, for which an underlying cause is seldom found and the treatment is difficult. This occurs more frequently in older white males. This tinnitus is described as ringing, cricket-like buzzing, whistling, hissing, or humming. It is usually associated with hearing loss and can be in one or both ears. Very rarely nonverbal auditory hallucinations such as crashing or train-like sounds are noted. This variety of subjective tinnitus is the phantom noise associated with abnormality in the auditory pathways, the cortex, and even the emotional limbic system.

With the objective variety of tinnitus, "real sounds" are

audible only to the listener. They include debris in the ear, the flowing of blood, or muscular contraction in the palate or Eustachian tube. These are typically described as pulsating, clicking, or fluttering.

Some folks have brief bursts of sound, but in general, the sounds come and go for the rest of the patient's life and is more of a medical nuisance than a true medical problem. One overdiagnosed disease is Meniere's, which is a low-pitch, roaring noise associated with vertigo, ear pressure, and gradual hearing loss. A rare cause of tinnitus, and one that doctors worry about, is a tumor of the acoustic nerve. These are unilateral and progressive, and unless diagnosed early, they can lead to permanent damage of the ear.

The treatment of tinnitus depends on the cause, if it can be found. In the older person with hearing loss, all that is needed is reassurance after the easily identifiable factors are ruled out.

Tinnitus frequently improves by decreasing alcohol, nicotine, and caffeine intake, better sleep, and decreased stress. Other treatments include niacin, B vitamins, zinc, ginkgo biloba, antidepressants, neuromodulators (Neurontin, Delcentin), craniosacral therapy, chiropractic manipulation, acupuncture (particularly in the external ear), and homeopathies. I have had some success with Otocom by Energique, a mixture of cloves, thyme, and echinacea that is dropped in the ear. When nothing works and the patient is disabled by their problem, a masking device emitting white or pink noise (the sound of rain, ocean waves, forests) is used. These can be inserted in the ear canal similar to a hearing aid. The use of inexpensive ear buds and listening to music can also help.

For more information, one can contact the American Tinnitus Association at www.ata.org.

TESTOSTERONE FOR VITALITY

A once neglected hormone, testosterone (T), is once again

coming into mainstream medicine. T is normally present in both men and women, but at much higher levels in males. Unless there is something dramatically wrong with the pituitary, adrenals, or gonads, T, which is minimal in prepuberty, becomes maximal in adolescence. Very rarely is there enough T, but the T receptor(s) are decreased. The most common T problem facing modern men is ADAM-androgen deficiency in the aging male. Androgens are a collection of hormones of which T is the most potent of the group of male distinguishing molecules such as DHEA or andriosterone. According to the older literature, these gave excitement, vitality, and even enlightenment. As we age, however, our testes produce less and less of this hormone. Moreover, some men earlier in life have this problem. There are numerous steps to normal T production. Initiating the process is LHRH (luteinizing hormone releasing hormone) in the hypothalamus, which stimulates the luteinizing hormone in the pituitary that encourages the production and release of T. In the male, the adrenal gland creates 5 to 10 percent of T, and is also under the control of the hypothalamus and the pituitary. The T is then carried by albumin and another protein, SHBG (serum hormone binding globulin) in the bloodstream. The former binds 60 to 70, and the latter carries about 30 percent. Only 1 to 2 percent is unbound to these molecules and is termed free T. It is this free T that is the messenger that accomplishes its fantastic life-giving and satisfying role. And what a job it does! Most people, including physicians, think of T just for the sexual benefit. However, the non-sexual health and antiaging benefits of T should make men at least know what their T level is when they feel they have lost their youth. If low, in light of their circumstances, consider adding this hormone simply for well-being. It is essential in both male and female, but since men have ten times more than women it is needed much more in men.

Brain function is improved. Like estrogen, there are T receptors in the brain. The proper amount of T produces better mental clarity, short-term memory, and mood. Those who were in a formal education phase of their lives, such as taking post-graduate courses or a new job, felt that learning was easier. Men who were subclinically depressed or dejected made a marked improvement in one to two weeks after treatment. At times it was subtle, and their significant other would report the development to me. Most informed me that they slept more soundly and their dreams were better.

Metabolism is improved. The more T, the less fat in our body. Not only does the obvious fat decrease, but also the invisible fat (serum lipids) diminishes. Triglycerides go down a lot, the total cholesterol some, and the healthy (HDL) cholesterol goes up slightly. Moreover, the lousy cholesterol (LDL) goes down a fair amount. Blood sugar and its three-month reflection of A1C hemoglobin gets better. Edward Lichten, MD, F.A.C.S., proposed that T is the cure for diabetes. Intra-abdominal fat, which is a predictor of diabetes and cardiovascular disease, is greatly reduced. The metabolic syndrome, with elevation of triglycerides, sugar, and blood pressure with a reduction of HDL cholesterol, almost disappears and its poor prognosis evaporates. The markers of inflammation, such as CRP and IL6, are reduced.

Muscle strength and mass is improved. T was the hormone of choice for athletes and bodybuilders in the past, and this drug was abused by taking massive rather than physiologic amounts of it. Taken judiciously, this compound will not only improve one's body composition by building muscle, but it better sculpts the body. Personal sports such as golf and bowling will improve, and if one is into endurance exercise such as biking, running or swimming, performance will be improved. If one were to train and observe a good diet, even better results will be obtained.

Heart health is enhanced. Not only does T help the risk factors for cardiovascular disease, but it also makes the heart pump stronger. Men who have had heart attacks and decreased cardiac performance, even some who were in heart failure, greatly improved. Men who had angina, chest discomfort on exertion, experienced improvement with T.

Bone density is normalized with T replacement. Not only will men have fewer bone aches and pains, but they experience fewer fractures. It makes a big difference with a fall in one's seventies whether you just bruise the hip versus breaking it, and all the problems that come with that unfortunate incident.

Sexual fitness returns. This includes erection, sensitivity, libido, performance, orgasm, and satisfaction. The psychological and social aspect of this may be overplayed, but T does help this important aspect of marriage that decreases as a couple ages. It is said that the more satisfying sex a married couple has, the longer and happier they will live.

General well-being comes back. It is hard to quantify this, but quality of life studies have shown improvement. Subjectively, men did not realize how low they were until they felt renewed life after T therapy. Decreased motivation, fatigue, low energy, and loss of vim and vigor were eliminated and a sense of well-being returned. They were more on top of their game. Most felt that they were once again winning in the game of life.

Prostate health may be improved. It is a myth that normal levels of testosterone cause prostate disease. If it did, we would see prostate problems in eighteen-year-olds, when T levels are high, rather than in eighty-year-olds, when they are low! There is a connection to T and the prostate, but this is from the breakdown product of T, DHT (dihydrotestosterone), which can cause prostatic enlargement and baldness. There has been some confusion in that PSA levels are increased by T and prostate cancer increases PSA. But that is where the connection ends. T does not even cause the benign enlargement. It is slightly controversial, but I have not seen a single male with worsening of the common urinary complaint of frequency and decreasing stream from T replacement. If there is a hormone responsible for prostate cancer, the literature suggests estrogen. Actually, it is the T/estrogen ratio that makes a difference. If it is less than 50 to 1, there could be a problem. T is converted to estrogen in the fat by a process called aromatizasation. So I occasionally check an estrogen level and, if high, give an inhibitor to that enzyme such as Femara, Casodex, or Aromasin. Of course it is mandatory to check the PSA level since it routinely goes up about 1 ng/ml within a month of T therapy. This is the new level.

Following the PSA velocity better detects cancer. It is suggested that if it increases more than 0.75 ng/mg in a year, it could be a marker of prostatic cancer. I personally discourage getting routine PSAs in men over sixty-five, since if they ever got cancer, they could die of something else, not the cancer many years later. If they went on to be treated for this cancer, their quality and perhaps their quantity of life would be decreased.

Real medical concerns with T replacement include erythrocytosis (too many red blood cells), the opposite of anemia. Erythrocytosis occurs less than 7 percent of the time. What does happen is that with T, the red blood count does go up slightly. Using the hematocrit as a guide, it is 3 percent, or with the hemoglobin, it is 1 percent. As long as the former is less than 52, or the latter less than 16, there is nothing to be concerned with. If these values are exceeded, I recommend "donating blood" in that the extra amount of the red blood cells makes the blood more viscous (thicker). Concommitently, I reduce the dose of the next course of T treatment. Acne has arisen in a few susceptible men, but this has always subsided with dose reduction. Breast enlargement has been noted in rare instances, but this also always regresses with dose reduction or with an aromatase inhibitor. Although described in the past with overdoses of T, I have not seen any liver or lipid problems, aggressiveness, or blood pressure elevation that was not there before or that came from other medical problems.

Testosterone level tests are necessary before T replacement. These are needed to not only correlate the symptoms of deficiency, but to determine the exact dose of replacement. In the past, salivary specimens, blood/serum levels, free T, SHBG, and morning fasting total T were obtained. After doing several thousand tests, I recommend only a random blood level prior to treatment and one a month later along with the new PSA and hemoglobin/hematocrit study. The lab gives normal ranges of between 200 and 1,200 ng/dL. However, these levels reflect the "normal" male population between nine and ninety-nine years old, not the ideal level for a healthy male who wants to feel and be his best! That value would be closer to what his level was when he was at peak fitness (which would be about 1,000), not just in the so-called normal range.

Incidence of testosterone deficiency is age dependent. The older a male, the higher the incidence. In 2006, the Endocrine Society came up with the consensus that there is no single value that would definitely correlate with the Low T Syndrome. Subsequently, guidelines have been established by the Second Andropause Consensus Panel. My view is similar.

Less than 250: very low
Less than 400: low
Between 400 and 500: borderline low

However, if the patient has symptoms with normal levels, I do further studies, such as SHBG, Free T, and LH. Sometimes all these studies are normal, yet the individual has symptoms. In cases like this, I suspect there could be a receptor resistance just as in Type 2 diabetes, or in Type 2 hypothyroidism. Here I treat the patient, not the lab test, by giving a therapeutic trial of T and following that person very carefully.

TESTOSTERONE REPLACEMENT

Testosterone replacement is not exactly the same as T treatment that a physician may do for HIV, refractory anemia, or muscle wasting disease. Replacement is giving the very substance of which the patient is deficient. The best replacement is with Bioidentical T. T has been used in human beings for over sixty years. The Nobel Prize for its discovery and characterization was awarded to a Swiss chemist, Leopold Ruzicka, and a German doctor, Adolf Butenandt, in 1939. T has been approved for treatment for over fifty years. Because of the possible abuse by athletes and others as "steroids," it is controlled almost as much as class A narcotic by the FDA. There are various ways to replace this hormone. Each has its advantage and disadvantage.

The easiest way is with a prescription gel, either Androgel or Testim. These cost over $200 a month, although they are covered by many insurance drug programs. Testim has a fragrance that is adored by some women and abhorred by others. Much less expensive is T gel or cream from compounding pharmacies. The cost of this is between $28 and $55 a month. Despite the drug companies telling men to use the substance on their arms and the front part of their shoulders, I recommend that it be applied to the nonfatty part of the groin. In that way, the T is absorbed through the same blood vessels to which it was naturally transmitted from the testicle.

Care should be taken not to put the T on the scrotum since the subcutaneous tissue would metabolize that to the harmful DHT, causing prostate enlargement and baldness. To take advantage of the natural diurnal variation of T, because it gives more vigor then, the morning after bathing would seem best. However, it can be used anytime of the day. It takes several weeks before a good blood level can be obtained and maybe as long as a month before the desired results are realized. The dose of T is as low as 25 mg to as much as 300 mg daily.

Another way of delivering T is by intramuscular injection, giving 100 mg on average weekly. The longer lasting T-cyprionate enathnate, or propionate, is being used now, but in the future the longer acting Nebido will be available. This will last ten weeks. Usually my nurse teaches the man or his significant other how to inject this fluid deep into the muscle. This preparation is cost effective. It takes four days to peak, lasts ten days, then drops off. Some men feel the peaks and valleys of this method. It also takes several blood tests at peak and drop-off (trough) levels along with the history of symptom relief to determine the correct dose and cycle of administration.

Perhaps the best way to have this vital hormone replaced is by the pellet. This method of management has been around for almost fifty years and, for me and my patients, this is the way to go. These are painlessly placed under the skin, mostly on the abdomen, occasionally in the buttocks, with local anesthesia. A commercial product, Testopel, or an identical, less expensive product from a compounding pharmacy are available and are easily implanted.[6] The beauty of this method is that the hormone levels stay good for about six months. Furthermore, this seems to be a more physiologic way of T delivery. In times of sex, exercise, and in moments of stress there is a natural increase of SHBG, and more of the T is absorbed from the pellet. It is literally a testicular bioimplant. With the patch, gel, or cream, it is erratically absorbed by the skin. With the shot, there is a roller coaster up and down. The cost of the pellet depends on the dose needed. Each pellet of T costs about $45 and the insertion about $200. A male might need 3 to 15 of the 200 mg pellets depending on his symptoms, age, and T levels. However, this is for six months and pales in price compared to the $200+ monthly for topical application, not to mention the daily chore of its application. Other delivery systems for T are the patch, which is expensive and causes a rash in 85 percent of the users, and the Buccal/gum product Striant that is replaced every twelve hours. These are seldom recommended these days.

In summary, T is a needed, not just wanted, hormone for a better life for both men and women. Although it can be administered in several different ways, the best for me and 94 percent of my patients is by the pellet. The cost is about $320 for women and for a man about $650 for six months of effective treatment. Some insurance companies pay for it. However, even if one has to pay out of his own pocket, it is a bargain, considering all the good it does for the individual in improving the quality, and the quantity of life. In almost 2,000 people I have seen fantastic results!

FEMALE HORMONE REPLACEMENT THERAPY

There is little question that hormonal replacement benefits definitely outweigh the risks of other diseases, particularly when bioidentical hormones are used. These are exactly like the hormones made in the ovaries. The human body knows no difference from these and what is produced genetically. The bioidenticals are derived initially from plant sources and crafted to be the same composition that is naturally produced by your body. Thyroid, adrenal, and sex hormones are available also bioidentically. Unfortunately, too many women in our country are not taking hormones because of the false concern that they may cause cancer. Medical doctors were hoodwinked by the media in 2006 to believe that taking hormones is risky. Three reports that show a minimal increase of breast and uterine cancer contradict the previous forty years of benignity in over 1,000 studies. Today, a woman who is age fifty and in good health could very well spend half her lifetime in a postmenopausal hormone imbalance and hence, be subject to increase of morbid problems. Female hormones are the only hormone abnormality in all of medicine that are not routinely replaced. If the patient has a low thyroid level, doctors prescribe thyroid. If she has low parathyroid output, doctors give her parathormone (Forteo). No physician would dare withhold insulin from a diabetic, but most physicians are not giving female hormones to those who need it most. Recent statistics show that less than 20 percent of postmenopausal women receive hormonal replacement and that most of them begged their physicians to prescribe them.

Research has shown that women who take unopposed nonhuman estrogen, such as from a pregnant mare (Premarin), that is, estrogen without progesterone, increases the risk of uterine cancer. However, this is a very slow-growing tumor commonly discovered because of postmenopausal bleeding and is rarely, if ever, fatal. I personally recommend progesterone if there is a uterus still in place. One needs only two weeks of progesterone every two months to prevent it. Better is using it as a nightly face cream. It not only retards cancer, but keeps the skin younger and enhances a good night's sleep.

Regarding breast cancer, statistically, one in nine women will develop this. . .if the patient lives to be 105. If a woman is in good health at age fifty and has not had breast cancer, her risk of dying from breast cancer is only 2 percent. This means that 98 percent of the time, she's going to die of something other than breast cancer, such as a fractured hip or cardiovascular disease (i.e., a stroke, which could be a fate worse than cancer). However, many women are blindsided by their doctor's false impression of hormones causing breast cancer.

I am not a fan of screening mammographies because there are too many false negatives and even worse, false positives, resulting in too many unneeded surgical procedures. That said, with mammography we *are* catching breast cancer earlier and earlier. Patients will have a 95 percent chance of long-term survival. A better way to detect the disease is through a PAP breast test.

There are other factors that cause breast cancer, which many women are not aware of. If a woman waits until she is thirty years old to have her first child rather than having her first child in her twenties, her risk of breast cancer increases 50 percent. If she is a little on the heavy side, her risk goes up another 50 percent. If she drinks, smokes, or eats too much fat, the risk of breast cancer goes up another 20 percent. On the other hand, if she decides to take a non-bioidentical hormone replacement and has been on it for five years, her cancer risk may go up less than 5 percent. If she takes a bioidentical hormone, there is no increase and maybe a decrease. A recent study shows she may have even less of a chance of an aggressive cancer if she ever did have a cancer while on hormones. A review article in *The New England Journal of Medicine* indicates hormone replacement impairs both the sensitivity and specificity of a mammogram in diagnosing breast cancer or recurrence of such. Stopping the hormones for two weeks before the procedure restores the accuracy of the study, and having a timely period once a year may be good for the woman.

The advantages of taking female hormones are great. Gynecological problems such as vaginal dryness, painful intercourse, decreased libido, vaginal infections, leakage of urine, and recurrent bladder infections are markedly improved. Uncomfortable symptoms like hot flashes, night sweats, mood and sleep disturbances improve within forty-eight hours of taking female hormones. As noted above, cardiovascular disease, in particular, heart attack and stroke, is markedly reduced by hormone replacement. Osteopenia and osteoporosis can cause pain if mild, and fractures in severe cases in women not taking female hormones. Moreover, hormone replacement improves memory and artery health, decreases brain cell loss, and can lessen Alzheimer's disease. Cancer of the colon, dental cavities, decreased vision due to cataracts, dry eyes, and macular degeneration occur more often in women who do not take hormones. Although not nearly as important to physicians, but very important to the individual, premature aging occurs more in women who choose not to take female hormones. Wrinkling of the skin, decreased vibrancy of the hair, and slow growth and cracking of the nails are common signs of estrogen deficiency.

Bioidentical or natural hormones are safer than the synthetics, as noted above. Most doctors who prescribe hormones use a combination of what the ovaries used to make in the form of estriol (E3) and estradiol (E2)—Biest. Others use the three natural estrogens: E2, E3, and E0 (Estrone)—Triest. I do not recommend estrone (E0), as it has been implicated in breast cancer. Additionally, the ovaries did make progesterone and a small amount of androgen. The androgen, or testosterone, is made mostly in the adrenals. It has been the neglected hormone in females. Testosterone should be included as part of a women's natural hormone formula. This is essential to normal sexual desire. It helps promote weight loss and improves the integrity of muscle and bone and exercise tolerance. Recently I have been prescribing Estriol as the only estrogen. It not only tends to prevent cancer, but also is anti-inflammatory. Soon E3 will be a patented drug used to treat multiple sclerosis, certain arthritic diseases such as rheumatoid arthritis and lupus, and in the future, allergies and atherosclerosis. Since it is available now for a fraction of its Big Pharma price, I use it almost exclusively when I prescribe estrogen.

The hormones are given by patch, creams, or the best, a subcutaneous pellet. They should never be given by mouth. If it is ingested, the major amount goes directly to the liver, where some unnatural metabolism could take place producing catachol estrogens that can potentially induce cancer. If God wanted women to take hormones orally, He would have placed the ovaries where the tonsils are! There are commercial patches of bioidentical estradiol, but none with natural progesterone and testosterone. Many compounding pharmacies mix all three of the hormones, costing between $30 and $60 a month. I instruct my patients to rub the cream on their groin, between the leg and the pelvis; not on the thigh where it can get absorbed into the fat and be metabolized by adipose cells into a renegade hormone, or on the vaginal lips where another transformation can take place, but in the narrow bony indentation on the underside of the hip. Then the hormones are transferred to the same blood vessels that the ovarian/adrenal products naturally used, with a fraction going to the liver and the rest into the circulatory system.

For the last six years I have favored the pellet, which is the size of a grain of rice and is inserted under the skin in a sterile and painless procedure taking five minutes. Many insurance companies are starting to pay for the pellet and/or the procedure. The hormones last about six months and if one would have to pay all out of pocket it would be about $300, the same as the cream and less than a prescribed branded hormone. Also, the pellet is much more physiologic in that circulating in our blood is SHBG (serum hormone binding globulin), which naturally increases at times of sex and stress, and more of the active hormone is released from the pellet as it is needed. Moreover, the SHBG reflects our natural bio-circadian rhythm with the innate early morning rise of the sex and adrenal hormones. It is like having a bioimplant of a real ovary and adrenal gland! A bonus of having the pellet installed is that it "cures" migraines. It is the sudden decrease in estrogen that triggers many of these headaches. This is why migraines are more common in women compared to men and that they are more frequent right before menstruation. The pellet gives a steady low flow of estrogen and is almost 100 percent effective for migraines.

What is most helpful in fine-tuning the exact recipe for a woman is her clinical presentation before and after her initial

BHRT. Depending on the patient's experience with the initial prescription, various components are increased or decreased until she is not only free of symptoms, but her body functions as it did when she was younger. Should the breasts become tender, we reduce the estrogen. Should she have fluid retention, mood swings, and/or migraine headaches, we decrease the estrogen or increase the progesterone. On the other hand, if there is excess hair growth, we decrease the androgenor and add Spirolactone. If the uterus is still present, there is always a chance for breakthrough bleeding, and if one stops the estrogen suddenly, there is a possibility of a heavy period. The prescriptive drug Lysteda will stop in three days any heavy period.

Doctors recommend antidepressants such as Serafem and Effexor for the symptoms of menopause; and nonmedical clinicians advise black cohash for hot flashes, chaste berry for mood symptoms, ginkgo biloba for memory and reversing senility, ginseng and pould arco for improving sexual function, passion flower to overcome insomnia, valerian to help one sleep, and various soy products that will function as estrogens to some extent. Phytoestrogens (plant source estrogen-like compounds) are converted into estrogen-like substances in the gastrointestinal tract. These phytoestrogens are xenoestrogens (foreign and toxic estrogen) and adhere to the estrogen receptor. It is the xenoestrogens that are thought to stimulate cells to produce abnormally and, in some cases, even to be the cause of cancer. Natural estrogens will diminish this by protecting the receptor site from these noxious estrogen disrupters. Xenoestrogens, particularly soy, will affect the thyroid receptors and cause defective thyroid function. So there is no joy in soy (see page 149)! Other receptor interference is caused by contamination by pesticides, hydrocarbons, and chemicals in our air, water, and food and on the skin. In our modern society it is most difficult to eliminate these from our environment.

Hormones should be started in the perimenopausal period

before women actually start menopause. A woman in her mid-forties who is having late periods, slight hot flashes, an increase in mood swings, a new sleep disorder, and a family history of early menopause should consider the need to start hormone treatment soon, rather than waiting for full-blown menopause. Studies show much less bone loss, an earlier improvement in lipids, and even a lesser incidence of Alzheimer's if the hormones are started while the woman is still having periods. However, better late than never. I have started an eighty-year-old woman on hormones so that she can have a longer and a better life.

Personality

There is as much variation in personalities as there is in differences in faces, and to compound the issue, it changes as to what time of the day it is and what one had in their last meal. Basically, nature, nurture, and many neuropsychological patterns form the personality that makes us the individuals we are.

After age thirty, the personality tends to be stable. As certain neurons in older age drop out, particularly in the prefrontal gyrus or the hypocampus, people become more mellow. Moreover, when some of these hindering intrusive thoughts leave us, we are no longer encumbered by too much confounding information and we can actually see the big picture, rather than focus on insignificant thoughts. Some experts feel that this is the beginning of wisdom. It is a shame for many of us that it happens too late. Sudden changes in personality frequently suggest the onset of a secondary disease process such as a mini-stroke. Drugs, toxins, and our environment can also change our personalities.

Teeth

Loss of the white protective enamel and discoloration of teeth occurs as we age. Not only do the bones holding the teeth shrink, but the gums surrounding them do as well, and the person is literally "long in tooth." The teeth are more brittle, thus breakage and loss of teeth are the consequence. Unfortunately, the refined foods, particularly the carbs, cause a change in our mouth flora causing plaque in the tooth/gum crevices and cavities in our teeth and jaws. The cavities in our teeth are easily fixed, but jaw lesions may require extensive dental surgery. To add insult to injury, the meridians (invisible energy channels) extend from our teeth to various organs and other parts of our body, causing them to malfunction. For example, if there is an anatomical problem in the left upper cuspid (eye tooth), our left eye will not see as well. As a country we have done well in stressing the importance of brushing our teeth. However, we add the toxin, fluoride, to toothpaste, which inhibits the good bacteria and harms our bones and brain. It would be better to brush our gums, thus stimulating them, and to *wash* our teeth. The best natural compound to use would be xylitol and baking soda. The former kills the harmful bacteria and encourages the good. The latter raises the pH in our mouth that discourages the twin demons of plaque and decay. If you are unable to brush or swish with this magic mixture of xylitol/baking soda, at least rinse your mouth following eating or drinking anything with carbs.

Bones

As we get older, our bones become more brittle because of the loss of minerals and protein, and the lack of exercise.

Until recently, I have encouraged my patients to drink milk. We now know that protein, particularly milk protein (casein), increases acid and, rather than retards, causes osteoporosis. The Atkins Diet or other high protein diets such the Eads Diet, may be more detrimental than beneficial for the bones. Diane Feskanich, in the *American Journal of Epidemiology*, tracked medical histories of 78,000 middle-aged women for over ten years and found that women who drank two or more glasses of milk a day were far more likely to have a broken hip than those who drank less than one glass a week![7] That is why the more dairy food people eat, the more likely they are to suffer fractures from osteoporosis.

Paradoxically, in older people the problem seems not to be the calcium as much as reduced protein, which is reflected by their serum albumin. For a variety of reasons, older people have poor nutrition. For better absorption, I recommend magnesium and strontium for minerals. Vitamins K, C, and D (10-20,000 MG/day) as helpers and Sodium Monophosphate. This natural chemical, which can be purchased at a horse feed store, should be used daily as a small pinch. It improves not only bone but tooth health. Added to the above mix is natural hormones and exercise. The exercise should not only be weight-bearing but torguing. There are several prescriptive drugs such as the biphosphonates (Boniva, Zometa) that cause problems like a rotten jaw or even an atypical femur fracture after four years of use. The recently released RANKL inhibitor, Prolia, is extremely costly and works poorly for this disease. With the above advised regimen, almost 95 percent of patients return to a normal bone density within two years compared to those on expensive, dangerous prescriptive drugs where less than 10 percent are cured.

Smell/Taste

The nerves that supply the nose with its olfactory sense begin to decrease around age thirty, and 50 percent of the sense of smell is gone by age eighty. Since taste is appreciated not only on the tongue but with smell, it is lost as well. Zinc deficiency, nasal/sinus infection, and allergies decrease our sense of taste. The overuse of salt reduces our response to it.

Skin

To sustain a youthful appearance, patients must address the systemic effects of age on the body. Long-term lifestyle factors, as well as anti-aging nutrients and hormones, will provide the most benefit to preserving or restoring youthful skin. Apart from the relentless ticking of the biological clock, much skin aging results from exposure to ultraviolet (UV) radiation from the sun, both UVA and UVB. Tanning beds are very harmful to the skin, producing lots of bad UVA radiation. To maintain youthful skin, it is best to avoid direct sunlight whenever possible, and wear protection when exposed. A good sunscreen is probably the most important long-term topical anti-aging preparation.

UV radiation and free oxygen radicals combine to stimulate the synthesis of collagenase, an enzyme that degrades collagen without stimulating synthesis of an anti-collagenase. The latter prevents collagen degradation. Eventually, this imbalance leads to the breakdown of collagen fibers in the skin's extracellular matrix, resulting in skin that sags. Sun also destroys some of the all-important immunity of our skin, making us more likely to develop skin cancer.

There are many health-based treatments that offer to improve aging skin, including masks, wraps, detoxifiers, and electrical stimulators that improve both muscle and skin tone. Visibly sagging and wrinkled skin signals much greater health hazards, such as undesirable cross-linking of tissues in organs and underlying tissues and cells. Since we are as young as we look, keeping our skin young will keep us young. The use of female hormones retards, and in some cases reverses, aging skin and wrinkles. The Langerhan cell living in our skin is a literal army tank. It waits patiently, and when a noxious infiltrating chemical, an invading organism such as bacteria, or a single abnormal cancer cell is accidentally produced, "Sargent

Langerhan" takes them out. UV light irreversibly harms this important immunity cellular form of skin protection. Hence, discoloration of the skin, infection, and cancers do occur more often if these cells have been damaged or destroyed by sunburns.

Rejuvenation of the skin can be accomplished by the fruit acid, glycolic acid. In high concentrations it is applied by a physician or prescribed for home use, but in less concentrated form. Phenol has been used in the past, but it has now been replaced by glycolic acid, laser surgery, and Botox injections. These are done by physicians and their assistants. The ultimate is plastic surgery, which if done, usually needs to be repeated every five to ten years.

HAIR

Hair is a wonderful appendage to our body. Not only does it protect our bodies, it looks good and is an attraction to the opposite sex—at least if it is on our head, face, chest, and perhaps other areas. When wet, this near-microscopic piece of our anatomy clings to hundreds of its neighbors, but when dry, with or without added enhancers, it has negative static electricity to volumize its appearance. Moreover it is amenable to various dyes and curl enhancers.

Our full head of hair will decrease as we age, but hair loss is much more common and severe in men. Every decade after the age of thirty, men lose 10 percent of their hair on average. That is 30 percent of men over forty, 60 percent of men over sixty, and 80 percent of men over eighty. More important, the younger the individual when the hair is lost, the more significant it is to them personally. Hair loss is a genetic predisposition inherited from *both* parents. In addition to genetics, hormones, too much sunlight, trauma, and harsh chemicals can influence the incidence and rapidity of hair loss. Stress, a change in thyroid, or sex hormones can alter growth and cause hair loss.

The specifics of hair growth and loss is that hair normally grows in two- to six-year cycles. Anagen, the growing phase, lasts two to five years; catagen, the regression phase, lasts two to three weeks; and telogen, the resting phase, lasts three to four months. At any one time, hair is always falling out. In male pattern baldness, the cycles do change, with anagen reduced to only six to eight weeks and telogen lasting for years. Over the years, hair becomes progressively thinner, finer, shorter, and less pigmented. On the scalp initially this appears as thinning and later, balding. This is noticed by the patient with more hair on the pillow in the morning, more in the shower drain and hairbrush. If the individual or the doctor were to look at the hair, he would see a small club at the end of the hair indicating that this is the resting, or telogen phase, an indication that the follicle is simply resting and will regenerate.

There are three letter presentations of balding; one, an O on the vertex, the top of the crown; another, more typical pattern is an M, with the mid part of the M pointing to the nose. This is called bitemporal recession. Lastly, the anterior pattern where a C shape referred to as anterior mid-scalp hair loss. As the hair loss continues, the front and back meet and there is just an edge of hair above the ears and around the back of the head. One way to tell if we are winning or losing the game of hair loss is the "pull test." Pull a lock of hair between your thumb and finger. Any more than one hair left in your fingers indicates you are losing. But look at the end that was in the scalp and if there is a little bulb on it, your hair will grow back. At this time one cannot predict when, but when it does, it will be more luxurious than before!

In the twenty-first century, there are options for treating baldness, including an aggressive surgical treatment with hair transplants, scalp reduction, and rotation flaps. These options are very effective, but they are fairly expensive and for the most part, not paid for by third-party payers. There are also hairpieces, hair weaves, hair enhancers (shampoos, sprays, mousses), camouflaging (Derm Blend, which colors both the hair and the scalp), and approved medical therapies. The latter includes Propecia and Avodart which is taken orally, and Rogaine, which is applied topically. Another topical product, Latisse (bitmatoprost), is used for eyelashes, brows, and may help the scalp. For each hair that grows naturally, two or three will replace it, although it takes two months to see the results. If treatment stops, the new hair will fall out. The increasing acceptance of a bald pate, as I have frequently observed, negates, at least for me, hair loss.

Canities is the technical term for graying of hair or, specifically, when the melanocytes (pigment producers) in the hair follicles produce less than a normal amount of pigment. Graying occurs independently of hair color and gender, but it varies with ethnicity. On average, in Caucasians, graying begins at age thirty-four, in Asians, at age thirty-seven, and in African Americans, at age forty. With Caucasians, the "50 percent rule" applies: Fifty percent of the population starts graying at fifty years of age. In men, the first gray hair appears on the chin whiskers, then the rest of the beard, followed by the scalp (usually at the temples), and then the pate.

Graying is a secondary result of a progressive decline in the number and the function of the melanocytes of the hair follicles. As time goes on, the melanocyte reservoir decreases in the ability to repopulate new pigmented hair. The average hair follicle produces only between seven and fifteen cycles of pigmented hair before it becomes too old to make pigment. This allows approximately fifty years of pigmented hair growth. In general, for every ten years after that, there is a 10 percent decrease of melanocyte production.

Gray hair is permanent. However, it may transiently darken, following some inflammatory processes, and there may be temporary intermittent bursts of pigmented hair. There are drugs that not only grow more hair, but make the hair darker, such as the antihypertensive, Minoxidil. Copper is also said to turn hair darker. Biotin increases hair's general health.

Premature graying may be caused by autoimmune diseases (pernicious anemia), thyroid disease, and nutritional deficiencies. It is associated with heart disease and osteoporosis. It is more than an old wives' tale that one's hair may turn completely white within a brief period of time following physical or emotional stress. There is a hereditary form of gray hair that causes a tuft of white hair, usually in the front. A family named for this feature, the Whitlocks, emigrated from England to America, and you can see their descendants that spot America.

Three Theories of Aging

The Telomerase Theory

The Telomerase Theory of Aging holds a real promise for life extension. Telomerase is now being dubbed the immortality enzyme. A telomere, as noted earlier in the book, is a piece of genetic material attached to the end of each chromosome, and it looks like the end of a shoelace. The cell's aging is characterized by the ever so slight shortening of the telomere with each cell division until it disappears. Then the cell can no longer divide, and at the end of its finite life, it dies. In the *Journal of Science*, studies on human cells show that a decreasing level of this enzyme leads to a gradual demise of chromosomes that ultimately stop cell division. At least in a test tube, we can now create immortal human cells by preventing the telomeres from shortening through control of the enzyme telomerase.

The Free Radical Theory

Although first proposed by Dunham Harman, MD, in 1959 at the University of Nebraska, the free radical concept was not widely accepted until the mid 1990s. Free radicals are very unstable organic compounds that seek out the chemicals of which our body is structurally made, as well as other internal pathways of life. Examples of this include the fats, which are then more rapidly incorporated into the plaque lining of our blood vessel walls. This causes the DNA, the genetic makeup of our bodies, to be altered and damaged, causing not only aging, but cancer. These free radicals are generated in the normal process of oxygenation and respiration. Our biochemical makeup is such that natural antioxidants neutralize these extra products of combustion like water putting out a fire. When there is excessive oxidation, our natural processes are overwhelmed and the extra free radicals do damage to our tissues and other natural substances in our body. To add insult to injury, we produce free radicals naturally from doing our regular business of living and energizing our body (eating, digesting, metabolizing). How we prepare our food also makes a big difference in the amount of free radicals or pro-oxidants we ingest. The consumption and absorption of toxins in our water and in the air we breathe (smog, carbon dioxide, pesticides, and cigarette smoke) do further harm. Another recent development for the human race is in the depletion of the ozone layer, which allows cosmic radiation to do more bodily harm than in the past.

As we age, the body sustains accumulative damage from oxidation. Our ability to neutralize the free radicals by the defending antioxidant buffers diminishes greatly. We have natural, built-in antioxidizing products that are composed of enzymes (gluthiothione, catalase, SOD), vitamins (C, E, polyphenols, carotenoids, flavinoids), and trace minerals (selenium, zinc). The antioxidants quench the free radical fire produced in our body's furnaces as well as from external sources (cosmic radiation and toxins). Antioxidants scavenge the free radical particles and, if enough are present, effectively neutralize them.

The Calorie Restriction Theory

After decades of experiments, the late Dr. Roy Walford, a respected gerontologist at UCLA, documented that a high nutrient diet, where the subject borders on malnutrition, greatly prolongs life. This has also been shown in various other species, such as water flies, spiders, guppies, rodents, and chiggers. Both the *Harvard Alumni Study* by Dr. H. Lee, as well as the *Nurses' Health Study* by Dr. J. Manson, found all cause mortality to be reduced by 20 percent in lower weight subjects compared to those of average weight. According to Dr. Richard Weinbruch, in a review article in the *New England Journal of Medicine*, the more one consumes, the more oxidative stress our cells are under, and the more rapidly they perish. However, after the age of seventy-five a few extra pounds, particularly if it is muscle, is healthy.

The Clock-Like Body

With my patients, I often compare the aging process to a clock. We are born with just so many tick-tocks embedded in our genes or given to us by our Creator. As we get older, the clock winds down as all clocks wind down eventually—even a nuclear one. But, just like the spring-loaded clocks made in the last 400 years, we should work perfectly until the last several minutes, falter slightly—and then stop. We should have 100 years of prime living before the clock strikes Old Age. To continue the analogy of the clock, starting at age twenty, when we reach adulthood, we cannot and should not turn the hands on the clock backward, although it can be slowed with knowledge of proper bionutrition.

Resetting the Biologic Clock

In the last 100 years, our life expectancy from birth has increased thirty-five years, but the maximum human lifespan has not changed much. Decreased infant mortality, better hygiene, and vaccines account for 85 percent of the improvement, while medical technology, with antibiotics and sophisticated surgery, accounts for only 15 percent. But caloric restriction without malnutrition slows aging and increases lifespan in both lower forms of animals and humans.

Aging is primary and secondary. Primary aging is the progressive deterioration of our structure and function due to the natural shortening of the cell nuclear telomere. Secondary aging is due to degenerative diseases such as cardiovascular (blood vessels), cancer, infection (immune system), and diabetes (metabolism). The more one eats, the more oxidative products are generated by the breakdown of food, particularly low nutritious carbohydrates. This causes chronic inflammation and metabolite alteration with the accumulation of injurious chemicals. Inexpensive Metformin has been shown to encourage weight loss, prevent, and even help treat some cancers. The downside is that it depletes the body's B12, which should be supplemented.

Lower body weight causes a slight decrease in body temperature and raises DHEA, both of which are associated with less disease. Of interest, rats that maintain low body fat by regular vigorous exercise in a running wheel, did not increase their lifespan like their sedentary mates who were just food restricted. In humans, the Atkins Diet did better, paradoxically, than a program of Lifestyle, Exercise, Attitude, Relationship, and Nutrition (LEARN), per a recent *JAMA* article.

Easily accessible biomarkers, such as fasting plasma blood sugar, low density lipoprotein, and blood pressure, as well as more sophisticated studies like left ventricular diastolic function, adrenaline metabolites, and insulin sensitivity were markedly improved in calorie-restricted people. Studies of European World War II survivors showed a marked decrease of coronary artery disease, which increased after the war and the return of adequate nutrition. Okinawans, with the largest number of centenarians in the world, eat 30 percent less than the average relatively long-lived Japanese residing elsewhere, and have a 35 percent lower incidence of heart and cancer mortality.

Although caloric restriction is recommended, it is hard to follow. A pill would be better. Metformin, 2-Deoxyglucose, and Resveratrol decrease serum glucose, insulin, heart rate, blood pressure, and adrenaline. Even intermittent fasting is better than nothing for life extension. The downside of caloric restriction is osteoporosis, anemia, muscle wasting, depression, and irritability. A moderate reduction of calories, a fair amount of exercise and decreased psychological stress will go a long way in allowing you to go a long way.

Pathway to Longevity

We must stay out of harm's way! (see page 197.) One must physically, emotionally, and psychologically stay out of risky situations. Stress leads to many ailments. The ability to achieve stability through change is critical for a long survival. To some extent, the sudden secretion of adrenaline, which prepares our body for fight or flight, may be good for us if, indeed, we have to physically fight or flee. Our adrenal glands are activated by our pituitary to produce adrenaline and cortisol. In our society, conflict that has to be resolved psychically rather than physically, is dangerous to our health. Since we are emotionally fighting, fleeing, or frightening, we are literally abusing our bodies during an adrenaline rush with the extreme revving up of our engine, without muscular motion. This is likened to racing the engine of an automobile for hours while the gears remain in neutral and the car not moving. Any mechanic will tell you that this will destroy the engine. This "emotion without motion" causes spasm of our blood vessels, raising our cholesterol and adding stress to our engine-like heart.

Excessive cortisol causes irreversible injury to our vital organs including the heart, causing coagulation, death of brain cells, and aging of our immune system. This may be the reason that the older we are, the more likely we are to have heart disease, dementia, cancer, and overwhelming infections.

Cherishing the one you love will add 6.5 years to your life. A long-term, committed relationship is achievable, but both partners need to give 100 percent. If you are in an unstable or unhappy relationship, get counseling to improve your situation. On the off chance that this does not work, when the children are raised (since you should be more committed to them than the spousal relationship for the sake of society), then break up. If a divorce is imminent, lean on loved ones, friends, and counselors to minimize stress and needless aging.

Love your neighbor; hate no one. People who have lots of friends, along with social and particularly church support, live longer and better. Loathing, holding grudges, and thinking bad of one's fellow man will take years off your life. Cynical distrust and even more, hostility, increases up to ten times the risk of having abnormal coronaries in young adults. Get enough sleep by hook (naturally) or by crook (herbs, meditation, or a prescription drug). This is seven hours a night or shorter with a daytime nap or meditation.

Having a pet, particularly a dog, can extend one's life. Walk the dog! It's good for the pet and even better for the owner. Do not be a risk-taker. One must avoid circumstances that could be dangerous, such as driving too fast, not wearing a seat belt, driving under the influence of alcohol or stress, taking chances by passing on the right, or not having enough clearance for left passage. You are twice as likely to be killed while walking with your back to traffic as when you face traffic, says the National Safety Council.

Although illegal in many states, some people still use cell phones while driving. Statistics have proven this to be extremely dangerous even if using a "hands-free" speakerphone. Texting while driving is comparable to driving while intoxicated. In other words, *never* do it.

Accidents do take their toll in maimed and dead bodies. The survivability in a potentially fatal accident is ten times greater in a large car (2,800 pounds or more) compared to a small automobile, according to Dr. Fred Rivara, a researcher at the University of Washington in Seattle. Smoke alarms should be installed in your home. While in a hotel, public building, or airplane, know where the nearest emergency exit is, in case of a fire or other catastrophe. Do not go out alone in a strange or large city at night. Take it easy in dangerous sports such as mountain climbing.

Do not ever over-drink alcoholic beverages or take mind-altering drugs. Do not have surgery unless there is no good alternative. Do not take any chances that may be dangerous, unless it is a life-or-death emergency and the risk benefit ratio is overwhelming on the benefit side. Be aware especially in poor lighting, of edges of carpets, thresholds of entranceways, or misplaced objects in your path. I am sure you can think of many other examples of staying out of harm's way. Of course, you also should know *not* to harm since in the big scheme of things, "what goes around, comes around." Staying out of harm's way retards aging.

ARISTOTLE SAID IT

Aristotle said it hundreds of years ago, and it still holds true today: Moderation in all things. This golden rule means to take nothing to excess. This should be your motto while eating, drinking, exercising, and playing. Resting properly is also necessary. We should consume the full (but not overdose) complement of supplements including vitamins and minerals. Try to stay as natural as possible. It is true, there is a science in nutrition, but it is still in its infancy. There are many other vitamins and essential factors in the wings waiting to be discovered, and consumption of natural products will contain these prime ingredients of life, compared to synthetics or partial compounds we think of today as healthy.

Avoid toxin exposure by staying away from pesticides, herbicides, chemicals in cleaners, paints, and various aerosols. Additionally, organic foods and un-chlorinated water and naturally fermented foods should be used to maintain a healthy internal "compost pile." Fresh air and exposure to proper light are also healthful. A positive philosophy for the mind and spirit, as well as appropriate exercise, should be included in attaining a healthy lifestyle to insure longevity.

EXERCISE WITH OXYGEN THERAPY

Live, work, and play in an environment that is as free as possible from pollutants in the air. Preferred environments include in the mountains, by the seashore, in a small village, or on the west side of your city (the wind blows from the west to the east 94 percent of the time). A fresh supply of filtered air in your indoor environment is a must. There should be a good supply of oxygen in the air. Indoor green plants are helpful, because they take in carbon dioxide and produce oxygen. The hemoglobin, which carries oxygen in our bodies, sends a message to the blood vessels through which the red blood cells are coursing, telling them to release nitric oxide. This increases blood supply to the tissues.

Dr. Manfred von Ardenne's research in the late 1970s reviewed more than 10,000 individual studies. He showed conclusively that there is a direct correlation between physical and psychological stress, aging, and low oxygen levels in the blood. Too little oxygen is bad, but too much is also bad. In the past, we physicians made too much of the possibility of oxygen toxicity, which affects only newborns and patients mismanaged in hyperbaric oxygen treatment.

As we age, we lose the ability to both absorb and "burn" oxygen. By age sixty, most of us have lost 40 percent of our ability to do this. Other factors, such as stressors (acute and chronic illness, surgery, and extreme exercise), have the same negative effect and contribute to the aging process. The less oxygen in our cells, the more free radicals are generated and the faster we age—it is a vicious negative cycle. When many doctors measure the oxygen in our blood, they tell us it is normal. But what they are missing is how well the oxygen is transferred to our cells.

A higher oxygen level in the lungs creates a greater head of pressure to drive oxygen into the lung capillaries. Exercise with oxygen therapy (EWOT) refers to a method in which one exercises while breathing concentrated oxygen; this markedly increases the amount of oxygen in the blood. Extra oxygen in the blood will actually push even more oxygen into our individual cells. Exercise moves the circulation much faster, ensuring a greater oxygen delivery. Initially, oxygen pressure in the veins rises as more oxygen is getting through on the venous side, but it is this oxygen that allows the capillaries to increase the transfer mechanism. Once the mechanism is fixed, more oxygen can filter through the capillary walls to oxygen-hungry tissue.

Here are the nuts and bolts for providing additional oxygen to the body during exercise: A drug-nutrient combination is orally administered thirty minutes before exercise containing 30 mg of vitamin B1, 100 mg of magnesium, and 75 mg of dipyridamole (an inexpensive prescription). Although not totally necessary, these agents will increase the uptake and utilization of the oxygen.

The conditions helped by this treatment include emphysema, circulatory disturbances, cataracts, senility, and arthritis. Getting started is as easy as joining a cardiac or respiratory rehabilitation program, where both oxygen and exercise equipment are located. If this is not available, or if you do not have a heart or lung problem for which third-party payers will cover the cost, you can inexpensively pay for it at home.

Oxygen is a drug, and a doctor's prescription is required. It is safe and your doctor should accommodate you. With diagnoses such as heart failure, polycythemia, and chronic lung disease with an oxygen saturation below 88 percent, insurance will pay. To validate this low level in a relatively healthy person, an exercise tolerance test is performed on a treadmill and, frequently, will determine the low oxygen defect.

An oxygen concentrator is better than bottled oxygen, and is easily rented or bought used for $250–300 from a medical equipment supplier or respiratory therapy company. Bottled oxygen, on the other hand, is cheaper in initial cost and readily available from local welding or medical supply companies, which can supply the gauge, tubing, and mask required.

The deliverer will place it next to your exercise equipment, and regulate the flow to five to six liters a minute. A re-breathing mask, which is best, has a little bag at the bottom to be used while exercising. It should fit over both your nose and mouth because both of these will be drawing in air. The storage bag ensures that there will be enough volume to breathe and will waste less oxygen, since the last of each inhaled breath and the first of the next exhaled breath is still rich in oxygen. This goes into the bag to be re-breathed. Although not for everyone, EWOT can rejuvenate most of us. The plastic hose, cannula, and prongs at most cost less than $10.

Nutrition

Albumin

Our nutritional status can be rapidly assessed by a blood test of serum albumin level. A value of less than 3.5 is indicative of malnutrition, says Ken Seaton, PhD, an albumin expert. He claims that this soluble protein is extremely versatile, playing a multifaceted role in our health. Albumin boosts the immune system and transports hormones, nutrients, vitamins, minerals, metals, and amino acids. Albumin aids in waste removal, cell growth, cell proliferation, cellular stability, electrolyte balance, kidney function, protein synthesis, immunoregulation, and growth hormone activity. More recent research has shown albumin to liberate nitric oxide. This relaxes our arterial walls, prevents coronary artery spasm, and figures importantly in preventing chest pain and heart attack. Albumin is also a mild antioxidant and figures into the production of HDL cholesterol metabolism. A blood test for albumin can be done routinely by your doctor. An even better blood test is the *prealbumin.*

Stomach Acid

Needless to say, we must eat healthily and properly. As we age, so does our gastrointestinal tract, and we digest fewer and fewer nutrients, which further impairs the healthy GI tract. The vicious cycle intensifies in that the less we absorb, the poorer our system works and the fewer nutrients are absorbed. Thirty percent of people over the age of sixty have less acid made by their stomachs than is normal. To make matters worse, doctors prescribe/recommend Tagemet, Prilosec, and Prevacid, which inhibits the cascade of ensuing digestive enzymes from being released, as well as preventing the gallbladder from releasing the beneficial fat emulsifier bile. Hence, the intestines themselves do not transport food substances as actively and as well as they age. As a consequence, some older people literally die of malnutrition; they waste away from poor nutrition. Their immune system becomes incompetent, and infections, some of which could be life-threatening, occur. If inadequate acid is the problem, it may help to take one or two OTC Betaine HCL 635 mg capsules at the beginning of a meal.

HEARTBURN

Heartburn results from the backing up (reflux) of stomach acid into the lower part of the esophagus. There is a valve called the gastroesophageal sphincter, which becomes so impaired it cannot keep the stomach contents where they belong. This is medically termed gastroesophageal reflux disease (GERD). It occurs in varying degrees in as much as 15 percent of all people.

Treatment consists of eating frequent small meals, not exercising on a full stomach, elevating the head of the bed by placing four-inch blocks under the feet of the headboard, and never lying down until two hours after eating a meal. Staying away from foods that dilate the bottom of the esophagus, such as chocolate, caffeine, alcohol, and onions, is advised.

Drugs such as Cialis and NSAIDS can cause reflux. The use of calcium products such as Tums is beneficial. Additionally, medications such as Reglan and Bethanechol, which keep the bottom of the esophagus closed, can help. One may decrease acid in the stomach by use of the nonprescription healthy drug Tagamet (Cimeladine) (200 to 400 mg one hour before meals), or the prescription drugs Pepcid, Axid, and Zantac.

Perhaps the best medications are the proton pump inhibitors. The first one was Prilosec, the next was Prevacid, and the most recent is Actifed. These are perhaps the best, but also the most expensive. The rational for treating GERD is not just the relief of symptoms, but to prevent the complications of esophageal stricture, in which the esophagus has to be manually dilated periodically with a forceful balloon. The other problem is that too much acid reflux for too long causes Barrett's esophagus, a forerunner of cancer. Barrett's is diagnosed by a procedure called an esophagoscopy, in which the doctor not only looks down your esophagus, but also does a biopsy.

Better Eating

Eating slowly and comfortably in nice surroundings brings additional efficiency to the digestive process. It is important to have a change in your mental state before you eat. This involves not merely sitting down at the table, but slowing your brain down as well. This is done almost automatically when we give thanks before we eat, but it can also be done by listening to music or having a glass of wine.

More than just eating properly, more protein, vitamins, and minerals need to be consumed as we age. Occasionally, we may have indigestion, bloating, and gas after eating, indicating decreased stomach acidity. If acid and/or enzymes are deficient, betaine HCL and/or enzymes (pepsin, lipase, and protease) can be taken in varying amounts with meals. Also, do not dilute your stomach acids by drinking water with meals. Plant-based enzymes seem to work better than those taken from animals. Eating organic raw vegetables and fruit also supplies us with their natural enzymes and are free of preservatives. A colleague of mine says, "If it is not raw, do not eat it at all." Go easy on grains, as they are acid producers and more caloric.

Remember that the end of the small intestine and the large intestine are our personal "compost pile." For proper preparation of compost, we need quality materials, including food, enzymes, and good fermentation. The latter is supplied by friendly bacteria. Antibiotic usage, knowingly or not, such as in meat, whose host were given these to produce better flesh, kill the friendly bacteria in our intestines. Additionally, chlorinated water will also lower the bacterial count. As noted earlier, one can repopulate one's intestines with live culture yogurt, kiefer, or probiotics. When we have the proper balance of intestinal flora, our internal plantation ensures against its invasion of yeast, bacteria, and viruses. The combination of a good bacterial growth and healthy fibrous foods (prebiotics) produces essential vitamins, stimulates our entire digestive system, and maintains our vital immune and hormonal balance.

Frequent small meals are better than two or three meals a day. The recommendation is for six a day, with the last at least three hours before sleep. This keeps the proper blood sugar level and tends to prevent fat accumulation. The GI tract, when it is full, actually burns more calories while it is working. Also you will not be famished before your next meal, and consequently you will eat less.

ENZYMES

Enzymes are protein substances required for every chemical reaction in the body and are found in all living things. At least 5,000 enzymatic pathways are known. In humans, they fall into three categories: food enzymes, which are found only in raw food and start digestion with consumption; digestive enzymes, which are produced mainly in the pancreas and break down proteins, fats, carbohydrates, and metabolic enzymes run the biological machinery necessary for our metabolism.

In the mid-1940s, "The Law of Adaptive Secretions of Digestive Enzymes" came into vogue. This indicated we only have a certain amount of the life force of digestive and metabolic enzymes. When these are exhausted, the end of life is close. German studies found that salivary enzymes in young adults were thirty times stronger than in older people. Animals who consume raw food have a pancreas one-third as large as ours based on body weight. Thus, by eating cooked food, which inactivates the enzymes, our pancreas must work harder and we run out of this life force sooner.

For centuries, humans unknowingly improved their enzyme potential by eating fermented foods. These were predigested by their own inherent enzymes. Examples are yogurt, kiefer, vinegar, sauerkraut, and some cheeses. Uncooked foods contain enzymes that correspond to its composition; lipase for fatty foods (nuts and dairy products), amylase for carbs (grains), and protease for protein (meats). Raw milk contains thirty-five separate enzymes, 90 percent of which are destroyed by pasteurization.

When taking enzymes, I suggest plant enzymes rather than those from animal sources, because animal enzymes operate only in the alkaline range, whereas plant enzymes work in a wide range of pH. Plant enzymes start working in the stomach, which is naturally acidic, and continue in the small intestine, which initially is alkaline. Animal enzymes work only in the small intestine. The more digested food is in our stomach, the less work is required for the pancreas.

For decreasing the inflammatory process in acute trauma, I recommend bromelain or papain; for preventing blood clots, nattokinase; and for treating allergies, bromelain. For best results, these enzymes should be taken *with* food. Enzymes should be considered at all ages when we are ill or take antibiotics, but routinely when we reach the age of eighty.

The Magic Injection—A Safe Steroid

Over the almost half century I have been doctoring, I have injected thousands of patients with local pain syndromes, using dozens of medications. I have injected into nerve roots, trigger/tender points, joints, tendon insertions, and even into the spinal canal. In the last twenty-five years, I have used Sarapin as part of a healing, pain-relieving cocktail. Although other specialists will give similar injections, including pain specialists, orthopedists, rheumatologists, and prolotherapists, my medicines and techniques seem to work better.

Prolotherapy, which has been used for over sixty years, heals tendons, joints, and muscles through the injection of curative substances, of which an irritant initiates the therapeutic process by the proliferation of new cells. It is also called sclerotherapy because it hardens limp tissue. Proliferants used in prolotherapy are substances that lead to new collagen formation. Collagen is the naturally occurring protein in the body that makes up ligaments and tendons. Prolotherapy solutions help strengthen these structures by initiating the first step in the wound-healing cascade, local inflammation. Once the inflammation has begun, fibroblasts are stimulated. These are the cells that make the collagen. New collagen is produced, making the ligaments and tendons stronger and tighter. A newer version of this is PRPC (plasma-rich platelets injection) and is FDA approved but not insurance paid. This procedure costs $1,000 for what I charge ($50) for a magic injection. The solution I now employ contains Serapin from the pitcher plant and 50 percent glucose as the proliferant. No cortisone is used because the inflammatory process is therapeutic—the steroid (cortisone) is anti-inflammatory and would therefore impede the process.

The pitcher plant (Sarracenia purpurea) is also known as Eve's Cup, Fly Catcher, Huntsman's Cup, and Water Cup. It looks like a pitcher or water jug. Like the Venus flytrap, it catches and "eats" small bugs. The pitcher plant has been used for stomach and digestive problems, for urinary tract disorders, and formerly as a cure for smallpox. Because it has not been used medicinally for several millennia, it has not been evaluated by the FDA for safety, purity, or effectiveness. All potential risks and/or advantages of the pitcher plant may not be known, but I still have found this to be an excellent and extremely safe medicine.

Sarapin is a biological medicine—which means that it is derived from that which is naturally occurring (that is, the pitcher plant). It works by stopping pain signals and initiates healing in the nerves. It does not affect any other nerve or motor functions as local anesthesia such as Lidocaine does.

Research published by Bernard Judovich, MD, used this preparation in over 5,000 patients and found it to be almost a miracle drug. Toxicity tests on Serapin published by William Bates, MD, in the *Ohio State Medical Journal* revealed that it was harmless, and no evidence of tissue coagulation or sclerosis could be found. Because it is an alkaline extract, which releases an ammonium ion from the organic matrix, it was theorized that this was the active ingredient in the solution. It is now known that this ion does affect nerve conduction, but Serapin does more than that. Perhaps the plant's special amino acid content, because of the organisms it ingests, created an unidentified biological fraction of the plant. And perhaps that fraction is the active ingredient along with the ammonium molecule. We know the C fibers in the nerve carry the pain sensation, and this chemical tells them not to. Acute pain is a useful mechanism for us to realize that something is wrong, but once that "something wrong" has been identified and there is no easy fix, then quieting these C fibers makes sense. Sarapin does not do only that, but it also initiates the healing process.

Science will probably never know the true mechanism of action because Sarapin lacks profitability and marketing dollars. As a biological medicine that has been in use for over seventy years, Sarapin cannot be patented. As a result, it can be made and sold on the open market without the huge price markups that are afforded to patent-protected medicines contributing to degenerative processes.

THE TIME OF YOUR LIFE

Time is defined as a continuous period measured by an instrument like a watch, clock, or calendar. Our culturally conditioned lifestyles are superimposed on our ancient genes.

In that ancient time, man had minimal things to do and a lot of time to do them. This causes time urgency, which prematurely and painfully kills. Twenty-first-century technology entices us to multitask with smartphones, computers, less physical work, and artificial light. We have become unwitting participants in our own undoing.

The sooner we intervene and do what is natural for our genes, the sooner we will be happier, living healthier and longer. The frustration of time causes not only harm to us, but damages happy and healthy relationships with family and friends. People are time stressed with multitasking, as well as by focusing externally on their next goal during their current task. Not only is it unenjoyable, but they compete against others as well as themselves to do things faster and better. When they are not overly productive, they become anxious. Only frenetic work reduces their anxiety, with a cost of too little sleep, exercise, and self-compassion. Overeating, alcohol consumption, and prescription drugs are their remedy and, subsequently, their enemy for decreasing their anxiety.

Initially, the excitement of the adrenaline rush, financial compensation, recognition, higher status, and the feeling of power can entice a workaholic or a super-mom. Later, they realize they might be the victim rather than the victor in the situation. Unfortunately, many people don't know the cost of their dysfunction until disease sets in. Adrenal fatigue, depression, cardiovascular disease, fibromyalgia, and decreased immunity can be the result.

Adrenal fatigue, for which there is no quick fix except with a life coach, a compassionate physician, and an understanding significant other, may be cured in six months for mild cases, nine months for moderate cases, and eighteen months for severe cases. With good time management, patients can keep their professional, familial, and personal sanity. The first step is to acknowledge there is a problem. Establish boundaries, like specific days to come home early, as well as overestimating rather than underestimat-ing time in doing a task. Do what makes you happy. With effort, you can stop your aggravated life of fighting the clock, a losing battle that creates a less enjoyable life and actually steals time from your life. In addition, "on the seventh day, thou shalt rest" (see Genesis 2:2). Give yourself a break on the Sabbath.

The Secret of The Secret

We are powerful beings who, with thought and deed, can create and destroy others as well as ourselves. We will never help our universe or ourselves by focusing on the negative. We create many of our diseases with over-observation and focus on our problems. Obsessing over an issue gives reality to it, amplifying the problem and making it worse.

Psychoneuroendoimmunology is a combination of many fields of study. Through this, evidence has given proof to the theory that negative emotions and thought processes upset the delicate balance of health. In other words, toxic thoughts are detrimental to our well-being! Negative thoughts have been found to acutely and chronically cause our bodies to overproduce cortisol, a hormone that is produced under stress, as well as adrenaline and insulin.

All of these "stress hormones" are able to give us the extra burst of energy needed to adeptly get out of harm's way in an emergency situation. However, in this stressful modern world of too much misinformation, overwhelming technology, an abundance of unhealthy foods, and the demands on our daily lives, these hormones are produced in excess.

Fortunately, human beings have the tools they need to modify their thoughts and behaviors to help them reduce the effects of these stressors on their bodies. The Australian author, Rhonda Byrne, wrote the book *The Secret* and produced a movie by the same name. These gave a new spin to the subject of thought modification. Affirmations (positive thoughts) have been around for centuries. My mentor of fifty years, Emile Coue, founded a psychotherapy method known as Coueism, which is based on autosuggestion. This is the practice of repeating a mantra, which would consist of a positive thought by an individual.

The affirmative mantra that he taught me was: "In every day, in every way, I am becoming better and better." Norman Vincent Peale, the author of *The Power of Positive Thinking*; Deepak Chopra, author of *The Spiritual Laws of Success*; and Tony Robbins, promoter of neurolinguistic programming, have said the same things in different ways. Byrne, who appeared on the talk shows *Oprah* and *Ellen*, wants to enlighten us as she did herself several years ago, when she was down and out. "Ask, Believe, and Receive" and "If You Believe It, You Can Achieve It" are her underlying pieces of advice. Being grateful for what we have attracts even more good. Praying for something (or someone) is easy in the Judeo-Christian ethic. "We reap what we sow" is an obvious maxim. The laws of attraction do create a better result through the right thoughts. By changing our thoughts, we can feel better, and we can create a better life situation. We are profoundly affected when we open our minds to opportunity and then, when an ambiguous event does occur, it will be noticed. It raises consciousness to the possibilities that will get our attention for success.

Eating to Better Your Health

Good health is not hoping for immortality, but being able to fully enjoy the time we have. It is about being functional as long as possible, and avoiding crippling, painful, and lengthy battles with diseases. We are living longer since starvation, poor sanitation, and communicable diseases were virtually wiped out for Western civilization in the last century. But now we are dying from diseases of affluence. If people were poor, they ate staple plant foods such as potatoes and bread. If they were rich, they ate meat and dairy products.

Animal protein, including meat and milk, can be harmful according to some new research. In particular, milk protein which contains 87 percent casein, causes an increase of cancer, cardiovascular disease, and other degenerative diseases such as arthritis. It is far better to consume the other 13 percent, which is mainly whey.

Although it is tempting to consume isolated nutrients such as vitamins from a multivitamin pill, minerals from a similar pill, and other supposedly healthy products such as lutein, lycopene, and carotenoids, it works better if you consume these naturally in whole food. It takes an orchestra, with these elements in the correct ratios, consumed all together, to create the wonderful music, compared to just an orchestra section like the woodwinds and later the brasses, each section playing the same notes separately.

The bottom line is to maximally consume vegetables and moderate amounts of fruit, with minimal dairy and meat products. As noted earlier in the book,, "If it isn't raw, don't eat it," but you can steam or parboil your vegetables, and of course, you need to cook meat products to kill harmful bacteria. Eat fermented foods, avoid preservatives (nitrites, benzoic acid), eat leisurely with lots of chewing, and drink little liquids with your meals. You will lose fat, decrease whatever disease you have, feel better, and live longer. A plant-based diet will allow you to be young when you are old.

6

Materia Medica

In this chapter, I have included information about vitamins and minerals. This is far from a complete list. Some entries go into greater detail, reflecting literature that is more recent, or not as well known.

Vitamins

Once upon a time, there may have been enough vitamins in our food that additions were not needed. This has changed drastically since their precursors have been leached from the soil. Then there is the change in humans' diet to more refined and less natural food, which lacks vitamins as well as minerals. Vitamins and minerals have been recommended by the government in the amounts needed to prevent deficiency diseases, but taken in larger doses, they will bring much better health (vitamin D is a good example). It is easier to write about these one by one as an entity and to define a particular vitamin. Nevertheless, one must realize that each is a factor in the larger equation of health and can function only in conjunction with their complementary biochemical or mineral partner, sometimes referred to as "co-factors." Individually, a specific vitamin is necessary, but it works better in concert with many other micronutrients. As noted earlier, the analogy is of a solo instrument in an orchestra that sounds good alone, but the ensemble of complementary instruments enhances the overall listening experience.

A vitamin is a substance essential for life that one cannot synthesize in the body. These phytonutrients are organic substances derived from plants, meats, and dairy products. The term *vitamin* was coined mistakenly seventy-five years ago from the phrase "vital amines" from ammonia-producing substances. But we now know better. These are minute amounts of an organic catalyst that cannot be manufactured in the body and must be ingested. The naming system for vitamins is inadequate, and it will be changed one of these days. In general, they were classified alphabetically. The confusion was made worse because as more vitamins were discovered, they were placed in subclasses such as B6, B12, D2, and D3. This poor classification leaves no room for vitamins discovered more recently, such as coenzyme Q10, bioflavonoids, and quercetin.

RDA (Recommended Daily Allowance) is an overworked, misunderstood, overestimated bureaucratic term that is close to worthless in modern concepts of nutrition. There was much excitement in the news media after a flurry of research in high blood levels of homocysteine and its link to cardiovascular disease, as well as an earlier concern for neural tube defects. In response to a public outcry, the government raised the RDA of folic acid from 200 mg to 400 mg a day. The dosage is given in two measurements. One is in avoirdupois weight, usually in milligrams. The other is units of activity (U or IU). These reflect the old biological assay of a vitamin. The research on these was done in different countries and led to different kinds of units. In more recent years. consensus groups have come up with international units (IU) that combine the varying units from the different nations.

Natural production of vitamins is better, I think, but I have not taken a big stand on the question of natural versus synthetic. If folic acid comes from sewage sludge or if bacteria are grown in a sterile vat, the body cannot tell the difference.

Natural products cause the rotation of a light shined through the crystal to the left rather than the right. This is sometimes levo- or dextro-rotation, or in a synthetic vitamin, half to the left and half to the right. This is called a racemic mixture and does not exist in true nature. Nevertheless, other than some amino acids and perhaps yogurt, it seems to make little difference in our metabolism.

PROPERTIES OF VITAMINS

Generally, a water soluble vitamin washes out of our system in a day or two. But fat soluble vitamins will last months. The question of whether to take vitamins with food or without food is of minimal importance. Nature wanted us to get vitamins naturally as we eat, therefore, it makes sense to take them at the proper time and in the proper amounts to supply the needs for your body's metabolism. Some vitamins are needed for the metabolism of food. Others are used in essential biochemical mechanisms. Most vitamins have antioxidant properties. Fats, protein, and carbohydrates are macronutrients, a storage form of energy and the building-blocks of our tissues. These are converted by the body into glucose, or simple blood sugar. The body "burns" glucose in the presence of oxygen to produce carbon dioxide, water, and an energized molecule. This oxidative process takes place in a microorgan in mitochondria cells. The energized chemical is a phosphated compound called ATP (adenosine triphosphate). This ATP is the electrical battery that powers our body as well as the energy transport system delivered downstream to cells in need of fuel. The byproduct of this oxidative reaction is the release of free radicals. These are molecules that are electrically unstable. The free radicals are used in destroying bacteria and combating a variety of microdisease processes.

When free radicals are not needed, however, they do mischief. The membranes around our cells, or worse, the DNA

Table VI-I
VITAMIN DOSAGE

The range of recommended daily amounts in a healthy person are:

Beta Carotene (Provitamin A*)......................20,000 to 50,000 IU
Vitamin A*..8,000 to 100,000 IU
Thiamin (B1) .... 10 to 100 mg
Riboflavin (B2).. 50 to 800 mg
Niacin (B3)..25 to 3,000 mg
Inositol (B8)..10,000 to 18,000 IU
Niacinamide (B3) ....150 to 3,000 mg
Pantothenic acid...250 to 500 mg
Pyridoxine (B6) ....0 to 250 mg
Vitamin B12 ....100 to 10,000 mg
Lactrile (B17) ....75 to 1,000 mg
Vitamin C...500 to 18,000 MG
Vitamin D*... 400 to 15,000 IU
Vitamin E*..400 to 1,000 IU
Vitamin K 1*...10 to 1,599 mcg
Vitamin K 2*...10 to 1,500 mcg
Vitamin K 3*...1 to 100 mcg
Folic Acid ....400 to 10,000 mcg
Bioflavonoids .... 50 to 150 mg
Biotin.. 200 to 3,000 mcg
Choline..500 to 2,000 mg
Inositol...500 to 20,000 mg
PABA.. 50 to 100 mg

*Fat soluble
Others are water soluble

in our cellular nuclei, can be ravaged to cause disease. If free radicals attach to DNA or switch on an oncogene, they can cause cancer. They can oxidize cholesterol to a particle that is rapidly absorbed by the blood vessel walls causing atherosclerosis or, in lay terms, "hardening of the arteries." Free radicals cause at least fifty degenerative diseases including aging, Alzheimer's, Parkinson's, atherosclerosis, and arthritis. These free radicals are neutralized or balanced with a system of antioxidant enzymes that include glutathione, catalase, and superoxide dismutase (SOD). These biCochemicals and their pathways have been so ingeniously constructed that they are preserved or rejuvenated in the presence of antioxidant vitamins. The antioxidant duo of vitamins C and E has been advocated for a long time as the most important combination in the prevention and treatment of degenerative diseases.

VITAMIN A

Vitamin A is fat-soluble and, in its natural and synthetic forms, is referred to as retinoids. In the diet, these are pro-vitamin As, from plants (carotinoids) and from animals (retinyl esters), and when absorbed, they are automatically converted to their most active form, alpha-retinol. There are rate-limiting steps that prevent the body from making too much of the active vitamin A. However, if too much of the precursors (carotenoids) are consumed, the benign carotenemia colors the individual. They can biologically use this excessive amount for months if they are cut off from this essential substance. Vitamin A plays a healthy role in the immune system (cellular and humeral), bones, vision, teeth, reproduction, and tissue repair.

Clinical application of mega doses of Vitamin A, oral retinoids or carotenoids is used for prevention or treatment of age-related macular degeneration, night blindness, acne, viral infections, and following trauma (surgery, strokes, heart attacks, and infections) for enhanced healing. In fifty years of doctoring, neither I nor any of my colleagues have ever seen a case of an A overdose, called hypervitaminosis A, some doctors overly caution their patients of this possibility. Older age, chronic liver problems, protein malnutrition, and kidney disease may predispose a patient to this problem. A person who consumes too much alcohol, has a liver problem, and takes large doses of beta-carotene may be also disposed because of an interaction between ethanol and beta-carotene. A cheap source of Omega 3s and vitamin D is cod and other light flesh fish liver oils. Folks who consume large amounts of this may have toxicity, however, vitamin A is not in other fish oil supplements in appreciable amounts. Many commercial foods are fortified with vitamin A, but not enough to cause problems.

Toxicity includes laboratory abnormalities such as elevated liver enzymes, high serum calcium, and elevated lipids. Also, GI symptoms can include abdominal pain, loss of appetite, diarrhea, and liver failure. The bones become painful and brittle and the teeth fall out. Neurologically, headache, weakness, confusion, and even coma have been documented. Toxicity can affect the skin (dry, itching, peeling), hair (loss), and nails (brittle). Acute toxicity can occur in taking more than 500,000 IU at one time. Daily intake of 25,000 IU for a month or, if predisposing factors are present, as little as 8,000 IU a day can cause problems.

The RDA is 3,000 IU for males, and 2,310 for females. The official UL (upper intake level) is set at 10,000 IU daily for both sexes to prevent toxicity. Clinically, I recommend 100,000 IU for no longer than eight days for acute infections and after surgery or trauma. For long-term treatment such as skin conditions (acne, psoriasis), I recommend 15,000 to 25,000, watching carefully for symptoms or lab abnormalities every month or so. Low serum levels are associated with an increased incidence of cancer and Alzheimer's as well as an increased mortality in AIDS. Vitamin A comes usually in 8,000 or 25,000 IU. Absorption is slightly better if taken with other fats.

VITAMIN B1 (THIAMINE)

Vitamin B1, a coenzyme, is a catalyst in the metabolism of carbohydrates, and it enables simple sugars to release their energy. B1 sources include leafy green vegetables, whole cereals, wheat germ, berries, nuts, and legumes. In its natural state, rice is rich in B1, but white flour and polished white rice are lacking in B1 since milling removes most of the vitamins. Rice husks, a byproduct of white rice, has much B1 as well as other excellent micronutrients and are found in some commercial products. B1 has a calming and focusing effect on the nervous system.

Even in today's world, we still see deficiencies in such diseases as alcoholism that produce abnormalities in thinking (Koraskov's syndrome), vision (Wernicke's syndrome), and nerve conditions (neuropathy). Although fewer than two milligrams a day are needed, diseases are treated with as much as 1,200 mg at a time.

VITAMIN B2 (RIBOFLAVIN)

Vitamin B2 is a coenzyme that serves as a metabolic catalyst in fats, proteins, and carbohydrates. Sources include dark, green vegetables, mushrooms, whole grains and cereals, avocados, green beans, spinach, and bananas. It helps keep skin and mucous membranes healthy. An abundant supply results in youthful skin, particularly around the nose and mouth. Scandinavian research has shown it to have been used in dosages 400 mg a day to alleviate migraine headaches and the symptoms of premenstrual syndrome.

VITAMIN B3 (NIACIN, NICOTINIC ACID; NICOTINAMIDE, NIACINIMIDE)

Vitamin B3 is found in lean meats, organ meats, fish, brewer's yeast, whole grains, nuts, dried peas and beans, white meat of turkey or chicken, milk and milk products. (Take note, niacin [nicotonic acid] is not exactly the same as niacinamide [nicotinamide]). B3 is known to assist enzymes in breaking down macronutrients into energy. Niacin in amounts greater than 500 mg lowers cholesterol and triglycerides and raises HDL cholesterol. It may also help in tinnitus (ringing of the ears). But in these high doses, however, it increases homocysteine, which is associated with an increase of cardiovascular disease, osteoporosis, and cancer. It may help the nervous system and maintain healthy skin and digestive tissues. B3 plays a role in the production of bile salts and in the synthesis of sex hormones. Nicotinamide alleviates the pain of arthritis in doses greater than 1,500 mg. Severe deficiency results in pellagra (which is rarely seen). The RDA is 20 mg.

Although available without a prescription, there are significant side effects. Almost all will get a flushing thirty to ninety minutes after taking crystalline niacin. Isohexoniacinate (IHN) and other slow-release products do not cause this side effect. Taking small doses of 10 to 25 mg daily and gradually increasing the dosage will diminish this annoying symptom. More worrisome is the elevation of blood sugar, liver dysfunction, peptic ulceration, increases of uric acid, eye problems (ambiplobia), and skin infections. In doses of more than 1,000 mg a day, periodic monitoring by a knowledgeable physician is recommended. Prescriptions of a slow-release niacin, alone or in combination with the lipid lowering statins, are available.

An increase in longevity from taking B3 is similar to that experienced by caloric restriction. Vitamin B3 makes up much of NAD (nicotinamide adenine dinucleotide) used by our cells for energy production when other sources are low. Nicotinamide, but not niacin, improves memory and is of use in the prevention and treatment of Alzheimer's disease and helps alleviate painful musculo-skeletal problems. Eating minimally for the rest of our lives means less energy production, less wear and tear, and most importantly less oxidative damage from energy production. NADH is available as a supplement (used for chronic fatigue syndrome), but it does not promote any significant levels of Sir2p.

VITAMIN B5
(PANOTHENIC ACID, CALCIUM PANTOTHENATE, PANTHENOL)

Found in brewer's yeast, liver, kidney, wheat bran, crude molasses, whole grains, egg yolk, peanuts, peas, sunflower seeds, beef, chicken, turkey, milk, and royal jelly, B5 is vital for the adrenal glands and its production of cortisone. It plays a role in creating energy from protein, carbohydrates, and fats, helping to synthesize cholesterol, steroids, and fatty acids. It is useful for a healthy digestive tract and is essential for the production of antibodies. It may help with arthritis since it has an anti-inflammatory effect.

Deficiency symptoms include a burning sensation in the feet; enlarged, beefy tongue; duodenal ulcers; inflammation of the intestines and stomach; decreased antibody formation; upper respiratory infections; vomiting; restlessness; muscle cramps; constipation; adrenal exhaustion; overwhelming fatigue; reduced production of hydrochloric acid in the stomach; allergies; arthritis; nerve degeneration; spinal curvature; disturbed pulse rate; gout; and graying hair. Although the RDA is 10 mg, the optimal daily amount is 100 to 200 mg in a B-complex supplement or up to 500 mg in divided doses. Many nutritionists feel that B vitamins should be given with each other so as not to cause a relative deficiency. I personally have seen no problems in giving just one at a time.

VITAMIN B6 (PYRIDOXINE, PYRIDOXINAL, PYRIDOXAMINE)

Vitamin B6 is found in brewer's yeast, sunflower seeds, wheat germ, liver and other organ meats, blackstrap molasses, bananas, walnuts, roasted peanuts, canned tuna, and salmon.

B6 metabolizes proteins, fats, and carbohydrates; forms hormones for adrenaline and insulin; and makes antibodies and red blood cells. It is used for synthesis of RNA and DNA, regulates fluids in the body, and is needed for production of hydrochloric acid. It can relieve carpal tunnel syndrome, fluid retention, and PMS symptoms. It helps asthmatics, and when used with magnesium, helps prevent kidney stones. Some nutritionists feel that some humans cannot convert pyridoxine to its active form of peridoxal phosphate and hence recommend B6.

Deficiency symptoms include greasy, scaly skin between the eyebrows and on the body parts that rub together, low blood sugar, numbness and tingling in the hands and feet, neuritis, arthritis, trembling hands in the aged, water rationing and swelling during pregnancy, nausea, motion sickness, mental retardation, epilepsy, kidney stones, anemia, excessive fatigue, mental illness, acne, convulsions, and cradle cap in babies. The RDA is 2 mg but the optimal daily amount is 50 to 100 mg (combined with a B-complex supplement). This is part of the vitamins triad (B6, B12, and folic acid) used to prevent and treat homocyteinemia. In certain rare genotypes, doses above 400 mg can cause neuropathy (disordered sensation).

Inositol

Vitamin Bh or inositol, is an organic natural chemical alcohol almost identical to glucose, which exists as myo-inositol in our bodies. Inositol or its phosphates and associated lipids are found in many foods, in particular grains with high bran content, nuts, beans, and fruit, especially cantaloupe, melons, and oranges.

Because it is produced by the human body from glucose, Bh is not an essential nutrient and therefore not a true vitamin. But in times of stress, our body may not produce enough for ideal body function. Greater amounts do help some medical issues. Inositol is involved in a number of biological processes, including prompting the stimulated insulin receptor to turn the nucleus "on," gene expression, serotonin modulation, and nerve conduction. Inositol is also used as the building-blocks of our cellular membrane, regulating intracellular calcium, and as a lipotropic.

As a lipotropic, inositol mobilizes fat, including cholesterol. We have used it in our weight loss patients with some success. It also rids the liver of excessive fat, which is almost becoming an epidemic due to our obesity. Because of fat mobilization and its insulin-potentiating effect, it has been clinically used effectively to treat polycystic ovary syndrome. Some preliminary results of studies of high dose inositol supplementation show promising results for people suffering from psychiatric problems such as bulimia, panic disorder, OCD, and depression. It also works directly (nerve improvement) and indirectly (better diabetic control) on peripheral neuropathy. Inositol has been used to decrease lithium toxicity and to strengthen hair, helping it to retain moisture. It is taken orally and is an ingredient in some shampoo formulas. There is no RDA for inositol, but taking one gram a day may be a good idea. Twelve to eighteen grams are used to treat the conditions noted above. It takes three to four weeks to see results. It is available in 500 mg and 1,000 mg caplets, as well as a powder in which 1 teaspoon is 4 grams.

VITAMIN B12 (CYANOCOBALAMINE)

As a young doctor forty-five years ago, I noticed my seasoned colleagues frequently giving B12 injections to older patients. These docs said their patients felt and performed better after such an injection. As a new doctor fresh out of medical school, I knew that this was just a placebo effect, since I had been taught that if folks ate properly, no one would need extra vitamins—

except the less than 1 percent of the population who had a genetic deficit, such as those with pernicious anemia. How dumb I was!

Now the National Academy of Sciences is urging older people to take additional B12 and not to rely on food sources alone. Since 1998, folic acid has been added to wheat flour to prevent neural tube defects in fetuses, but now there has been much more documented B12 deficiency in the elderly and much more dementia. Prior to folic acid fortification of wheat, B12 deficiency caused pernicious anemia. Now that there is excess of folic acid in our diets, the anemia is masked, but we do see one of the main consequences of B12 deficiency, dementia. Many older folks, because of a lack of stomach acid and/or because they are taking prescription medicine, cannot absorb even the minimal amount of B12 in their food. The recommended B12 blood value of greater than 1.50pmol/l is unreliable. I have been suspicious of this for the last decade since I read an article in the *Journal of the American Geriatric Society* recommending routine doses of 1,000 to 5,000 ug (*ug* stands for microgram and is one-millionth of a gram) of B12 in the elderly, since their deficiency was commonly undiagnosed.

What about reducing the folic acid supplemented in wheat flour? I believe folic acid should continue to fortify our wheat products to prevent birth defects. Also, importantly, it decreases serum homocysteine (a leading risk factor for cardiovascular disease), and by another mechanism, the incidence of cancer. The government should fortify foods with B12, as well. Until that happens, I will continue to give B12 injections. It can also be taken sublingually (under the tongue), or even orally at doses of 1,000 to 5,000 ug daily. Some folks cannot metabolically convert the oral, sublingual, or even the injected B12 to its active form. So many doctors in the know recommend the Hydroxycobalamine or even better methylcobalamine. It is extremely safe, very inexpensive, and whether coincidentally or causally, it improves vitality as well as helping the mind work better. Let's get on the "brain wagon" before it's too late.

B12 is red, and to determine if one is B12 sufficient, we ask the patient to watch the color of the urine. If reddish, the person has enough B12 with the excess B12 coming out, harmlessly, in the urine. If the urine is not red, we recommend taking the shots more frequently until it turns red, then increasing the shot interval.

As much as 40 percent of individuals over fifty do not have the needed mechanism to absorb B12. There are twenty-four steps involved in its absorption and activation. The first is the secretion of factors in the stomach, including acid, to start the process. Many people just don't have enough acid, or they may take acid blockers that inhibit this factor. Even taken under the tongue, many folks can't process it, so for them, receiving a B12 shot would be best.

VITAMIN B13 (OROTIC ACID)

There is not much information available about orotic acid. It has been used recently as orotate salts combined with such minerals as calcium, magnesium, and potassium. This is based on the work by the late German doctor Hans Nieper. Dr. Nieper's work has included these mineral orotates in his treatment of multiple sclerosis and other chronic diseases. His experience concluded that orotate salts were active transporters of these minerals into the blood from the gastrointestinal tract. The salts then separate from the mineral in the blood, allowing the mineral to be used to lubricate the metabolic machinery and leaving orotic acid available.

Orotic acid is found in a few natural food sources—for example, milk products and some root vegetables, such as carrots, beets, and Jerusalem artichokes. Orotic acid is a nucleic acid precursor needed for DNA and RNA synthesis. The body can make orotic acid for this purpose from its amino acid pool.

As long as protein nutrition is adequate, the body can carry on nucleic acid synthesis. Neither toxicity nor deficiency of orotic acid are likely a concern.

Recently, many exaggerated medical claims about orotates have been made by foreign markets and the U.S. alternative health industry. For this reason, and possibly other political-economic ones, the U.S. Food and Drug Administration (FDA) has asked for the removal of orotates from the U.S. marketplace.

Vitamin B15 (Pangamic Acid)

This is still a fairly controversial "vitamin." The quotation marks suggest that we are not sure whether it really is a vitamin. It has not yet been shown to be essential in the diet, and no symptoms or deficiency diseases are clearly revealed when its consumption is restricted.

Vitamin C

Vitamin C is the most widely used vitamin. It is also called ascorbic acid. It was the agent used to prevent scurvy in the sixteenth century. This vitamin is found naturally in fruits, particularly citrus, and vegetables. Its water solubility also means that excess amounts are eliminated through urination. Evolution has deprived humans of the ability to produce Vitamin C, but most other animals do manufacture it for their own bodies. The RDA is 60 mg, an amount designed to prevent scurvy. One-tenth of an orange a day or one-fifth of a lime will prevent the dreaded disease of old-time sailors, alcoholics, and individuals with odd diets. In thirty-five years as a clinician, I have seen only one case of scurvy. The dose of Vitamin C you should take depends on the purpose. It helps repair tissue, according to my colleague, cardiologist Daniel Levy, MD, who wrote the book *Change of Heart: Unraveling the Mysteries of Cardiovascular Disease,* Vitamin C also repairs the basement membrane in the endothelial cells, preventing atherosclerosis.

Higher doses may be needed following surgery and other physical and emotional diseases to which we all can fall prey. I recommend at least four grams (4,000 mg) a day but if you are under stress of disease or surgery, I would recommend six to eight grams a day. Some natural doctors give two grams every hour until diarrhea occurs, then stop. Scientist Linus Pauling, a two-time Nobel Prize winner, took eighteen grams a day for decades and lived to be ninety-four.

Research on Vitamin C has shown positive results in preventing heart disease, cancer, some infections, birth defects, and aging. Because it is water soluble, some experts advise taking half the daily amount twice a day. There is a controversy in nutrition concerning whether Vitamin C needs to be taken with bioflavinoids, as is found naturally in the plants that contain it. My feeling is that it can be given alone and that bioidentical C works as well as the natural. Some scientists feel that neutral sodium ascorbate works better than the acidic ascorbic acid. It commercially comes this way, but it can easily be made at home with equal parts of baking soda and ascorbic acid. Upper gastrointestinal problems can be stopped by reducing the dose to less than one gram a day, taking the dose with food, or better yet, taking Ester-C. It seems if one has a problem that really is vitamin C responsive, such as a viral infection, the dose can be easily increased to 20 to 40 grams a day without any diarrhea, but when the infection resolves, this dose then would cause diarrhea.

Vitamin D

Vitamin D is a prehormone that has two major forms, D2 (ergocalciferol) and D3 (cholecalciferol). Classically, vitamin D is obtained from sun exposure, food, and supplements. Just under the skin, UV light converts cholesterol to pre–Vitamin D, which is absorbed into the bloodstream where it travels to the liver then the kidney. In these organs it is hydroxylated each time to reach its active form, calcitriol. In the past, its major role was to increase the flow of calcium into the bloodstream by promoting absorption of calcium and phosphorus from food in the intestines, and reabsorption of calcium in the kidneys, enabling normal mineralization and remodeling of bone. In deficiency states, rickets can occur, particularly in children. Rickets can be remedied by sunshine and, in the winter, cod liver oil.

This sunshine vitamin does much more. It improves the function of the cardiovascular, immune, neurologic, and endocrine systems and independently extends life. To get the most out of this vitamin, it must be given in sufficient amounts, such as a daily intake of at least 10,000 IU, which is what one can get from the sun in a fair-skinned individual wearing a bathing suit without sun blockers between ten AM and three PM in the summer, assuming the kidneys and liver are normally functioning. Of course the downside would be an incredible sunburn with an increased risk of skin aging and cancer. The darker the skin by previous tanning or genetics, the less this essential substance is produced. So most of us have a deficiency of this miracle hormone-like vitamin. This is particularly true in the elderly, African Americans, those living in northern latitudes in the winter, most of whom have a real deficit of this molecule.

To assume that all of us have a D insufficiency and to take 10,000 IU, may be fine. To be more accurate and to ensure that we take the correct dose and not reach toxic levels, a blood test is advisable. According to the National Health and Nutrition Examination Survey, a group of researchers concluded that having low levels of Vitamin D was associated with an increase in all-cause mortality in the general population. The study evaluated whether low serum vitamin D levels were associated with all-cause mortality, cancer, and cardiovascular disease (CVD) mortality among 13,331 diverse American adults who were twenty years or older. Vitamin D levels of these participants were collected over a six-year period (from 1988 through 1994), and individuals were passively followed for mortality through the year 2000. Shortening of leukocyte telomeres is a marker of aging. Leukocyte telomere length predicts the development of aging-related disease, and the length of these telomeres decreases with each cell division and with increased inflammation (more common in the elderly). Vitamin D can inhibit proinflammatory overreaction and slow the turnover of leukocytes. In optimal concentrations, Vitamin D helps maintain leukocyte telomere length.

Lack of Vitamin D synthesis is a possible explanation for high rates of influenza and other respiratory infections during winter. The National Jewish Hospital recently published a study showing that there is a decrease of asthmatic attacks in patients who took 10,000 IU of vitamin D daily. Vitamin D has been shown to increase the activity of white cells, and it enhances the protective action of macrophages. Active Vitamin D hormone also increases the production of an antimicrobial peptide that is triggered by bacteria, viruses, and fungi. The fact that MS is more common in the higher latitudes suggests a link between Vitamin D and this disease. It is postulated that it is due to the immune-response suppression properties of Vitamin D. Early in 2010 another paper indicated that this vitamin decreases the incidence of cases and the exacerbation of Crohn's, the well-known autoimmune/infectious disease. The immune system needs Vitamin D to differentiate between your own and foreign proteins, especially in a subgroup of individuals genetically predisposed to various autoimmune diseases.

Vitamin D may both prevent and decrease the aggressiveness of cancer. Vitamin D plays a role in a wide range of cellular mechanisms in the development of cancer. A 2006 study using data of more than 4 million cancer patients from thirteen different countries showed a marked increase in some cancer risks in countries with less sun. Vitamin D reduced an individual's colon cancer risk by 50 percent, and breast and ovarian cancer risks by 30 percent. Low levels of Vitamin D have been correlated with breast cancer disease progression and bone metastases. A 2006 study found that taking the RDA of Vitamin D (400 IU per day) cut the risk of pancreatic cancer by 43 percent in a sample of more than 120,000 people from two long-term health surveys. Also in male smokers there is a threefold increased risk for pancreatic cancer for those in the lowest 20 percent of Vitamin D concentration. A 2007 study involving 1,200 women reports that Vitamin D supplementation resulted in a 60 percent reduction in cancer incidence during a four-year clinical trial, and a 77 percent reduction for cancers diagnosed after the first year.

A recent report from the National Health and Nutrition Examination Survey involving nearly 5,000 participants found that low levels of Vitamin D were associated with an increased risk of peripheral artery disease. The incidence of this was 80 percent higher in participants with the lowest Vitamin D levels. Low levels of Vitamin D are associated with an increase in high blood pressure.

There is a certain amount of evidence to suggest that dietary Vitamin D may be carried by fatty particles into and out of the cells of the artery wall and atherosclerotic plaque, where it may be converted to inactive form. Higher Vitamin D levels have been correlated with calcified plaques, but these are more stable than the "soft" non-calcified lesions.

I have found over 250 peer-reviewed articles verifying that Vitamin D lowers the incidence and severity of diabetes. Also this vitamin, perhaps because of its interaction with Vitamin A, greatly ameliorates psoriasis. I advise 5,000 to 15,000 IU a day with or without food, although its absorption may be better with meals. Some doctors recommend it in higher doses (50,000 to 100,000 IU) weekly or even monthly, but we were intended to get our Vitamin D daily from sunlight, so I advise daily consumption. The upper intake level of Vitamin D for children and adults is set at 2,000 IU. There have been published cases of individuals who have mistakenly taken 50,000 IU daily for two months without undue toxicity. Vitamin D overdose, however, can cause hypercalcemia, which has these primary symptoms: anorexia, nausea, and vomiting, frequently followed by weakness, nervousness, and ultimately, kidney damage, which may be irreversible. In my nearly fifty years as a physician, I have never seen such a case, nor have any of my colleagues.

Vitamin E

The two vitamins most commonly named as potent antioxidants are Vitamin C and E. Numerous studies have shown that the water-soluble Vitamin C is beneficial in that it rejuvenates fat-soluble Vitamin E. Many of the earlier studies have been done with natural Vitamin E rather than commercial Vitamin E. My research of the literature and experience with my patients indicates that a Vitamin E supplement by itself does not supply adequate antioxidant protection to neutralize the free radicals that cause degenerative diseases, including aging.

To obtain optimal health benefits from Vitamin E, a mixture of three other tocopherols (beta, gamma, and delta) and their sister, tocotrienol (alpha, gamma, beta, and delta), are required. Some of the functions of these Vitamin E fractions are similar, while others are completely different. When taken together, these various forms of Vitamin E work synergistically, as a team, to provide maximum benefit. If one takes the commercial form of Vitamin E, there is evidence that the effect of the antioxidant is not present. The difference between tocopherol and tocotrienol is a subtle change in their molecular structure.

Tocotrienol is able to move efficiently within the cell membranes and therefore is more able to neutralize the free radicals.

This may explain why Vitamin E found in foods is much more effective than the single alpha-tocopherol supplements. Hence, the broad spectrum Vitamin E is effective, whereas the isolated alpha-tocopherol is not. There is some evidence that indicates that alpha-tocopherol will decrease the effectiveness in the sister vitamin family. Moreover, like the statin drugs, tocotrienol has been shown to decrease cholesterol by a similar mechanism. They are shown to work like aspirin in decreasing the blood-clotting ability of our platelets and, like the drug Celebrex, to decrease inflammation of our joints, etc. Tocotrienol also possesses the ability to stimulate the killing of cancer through program death of these cells, referred to as apoptosis, leaving normal cells unaffected. In particular, breast and prostate cancer have been shown to be subdued by tocotrienol.

Although Vitamin E has an excellent safety record, studies indicate that the alpha-tocopherol alone without a mix of other tocopherols and tocotrienols is pro-oxidant rather than antioxidant. Therefore, I would suggest obtaining a full spectrum Vitamin E, available in most health food stores, or Gamma E. Far less effective commercial vitamin E is plain alpha-tocopherol that is found in multivitamins and sold by itself. Best is getting Vitamin E from nuts and seeds.

Vitamin K (K, K2, Menaquinone, Phytonadione)

Vitamin K gives protection against arterial calcification, Alzheimers, bone loss, cancer, and even aging! Although discovered in 1929, both Edward Adelbert Doisy (who died in1986) an American biochemist along with his Danish collegue, Henrik Dam received the Nobel Prize in Physiology Medicine in 1943. The new vitamin received the letter K because the initial work was reported in a German journal, in which it was designated as

Koagulationsvit (K from "Koagulations"). However, this fat soluble vitamin in light of the last decade of research has been shown to do much more than coagulate patients who have a low amount of activated clotting factors such as occurs in people who take the drug warfain (Coumadin), poor intestinal flora, malnutrition, or impaired liver function.

Normally as one ages calcification of soft tissues throughout the body such as heart valves, cornea, glands, and blood vessels occurs. Autopsies report 75% of folks over 75 have significant calcification and dysfunction of these organs! Dietary calcium is not the culprit causing this problem. The reason for this contradiction is that in response to a deficit of calcium in the blood, the parathyroid gland produces more of its hormone (PTH), which robs our bones and saturates soft tissues with calcium. Magnesium decreases the PTH output and counteracts the calcium bone loss. The action of vitamin K in the body is to carboxylate proteins. Carboxylation is an addition of a carboxyl group into a compound or molecule. When a protein is carboxylated, it undergoes a chemical conversion that changes its function. Vitamin K maintains normal coagulation, preserves bone, and protects against calcification by carboxylating specific proteins in the body. In the arteries, vitamin K is required to carboxylate matrix Gla-protein. If Matrix Gla-Protein (MGP) is under-carboxylated, then it is unable to perform its normal role in protecting arteries against excess accumulation of calcium, or inhibiting vascular calcification. Matrix Gla-protein is a calcification inhibitor that requires sufficient vitamin K to function optimally. The effect of vitamin K in carboxylating matrix Gla-protein is how it protects against arterial calcification.

Atherosclerosis is the leading cause of disability and death in civilized societies. Many factors are involved in its initiation and progression to include elevated blood pressure, sugar, uric acid, lipids, fibrinagen, Plac-2, Lp(a), MPO, homocysteine, smoking, kidney disease, and even non specific inflammation. These initially damage the inner arterial lining (the endothelium). To repair this damage, the endothelium produces collagen that contains MGA which forms a cap and macrophages that entrap oxidized cholesterol within the injury.

These endothelial collagen caps with their underlying cholesterol burden attract calcium through the MGP mechanism that subsequently accumulates calcium which forms a hard material resembling bone. This is why atherosclerosis is referred to as "hardening of the arteries." Atherosclerosis is the *soft* plaque before it becomes harden with calcium. Whether MPG allows or prevents calcification depends on its state of carboxylation. It is Vitamin K that carboxylates the MGP and inhibits calcification. Not enough Vitamin K then calcium is deposited. Calcification of the coronary arteries markedly increases the risk of myocardial infarction and heart failure. The same process takes place in our heart valves as we age particularly the aortic, which in addition to the other risk factors noted above has the highest pressure for the thinnest tissue of any place in the body.

A substantial volume of studies shows that different tissues need varying amounts of carboxylation for complete saturation and only minimal amounts of Vitamin K is needed to carboxylate (activate) the clotting factors. But much more is needed to inhibit MGA from calling in calcium to the "injured" site. So, insufficient vitamin K2 accelerates arterial calcification. A recent study shows that restoring to high levels of vitamin K2 reverses arterial and valvular calcification.

Jack LaLanne was an expert in all things health to include nutrition, but the science was not yet ready when he in 2003 he published his last book *Revitalize Your Life*. He used the precepts of the book to maintain his health, but his diet and supplements did not have enough Vitamin K. Due to this, genetics and his age, he developed Aortic Stenosis, and unfortunately was talked into valve replacement in 2009. This started his down hill spiral that twelve and a half months later eventuated in his death at age 96.

Vitamin K is as important in bone health as is Vitamin D. Bone is living tissue that is in a constant state of renewal. The maintenance of bone first requires old bone to be dissolved by cells called "osteoclasts." When the activity of osteoclasts is too high, large holes develop that weaken the bone and lead to osteoporosis. Vitamin K2 is a key to turning off excess osteoclast activity and bone degradation.

The holes left by osteoclasts are prepared for remodeling by osteoblast cells. The osteoblasts secrete a protein called osteocalcin, the synthesis of of which requires vitamin D3. But it needs to be activated (or carboxylated) by Vitamin K for new calcium to be laid down into the bone.

To reiterate, the calcium-binding properties of osteocalcin require vitamin K for two critical processes to the bone. It first protects against excess bone degradation (resorption) by turning off excess osteoclast activity. It then supports new bone formation by enabling osteocalcin to pull calcium from the blood and layer it on to the bone. Maintenance of healthy bone density requires adequate levels of magnesium, calcium, strontium and Vitamins D, C, and K. Without vitamin D, there will be no osteocalcin for vitamin K to work on. Without vitamin K, the osteocalcin that is produced will be inactive. And of course without calcium (and other minerals), there will be no minerals for the activated osteocalcin to attract to the bone for structural density.

The Nurses' Health Study followed more than 72,000 women for 10 years and found that women whose vitamin K intakes were in the lowest quintile (1/5) had a 30% higher risk of hip fracture than women with vitamin K intakes in the highest four quintiles. Another (seven-year) study in over 888 elderly men and women (Framingham Heart Study) found that men and women with dietary vitamin K intakes in the highest quartile (1/4) had a 65% lower risk of hip fracture than those with dietary vitamin K intakes in the lowest quartile (approximately 254 micrograms/day vs. 56 micrograms/day of vitamin K). In Japan it is approved by prescription to treat Osteoporosis.

Vitamin K has been proven to be beneficial for prevention and even the treatment of several cancers. These include Lung, Pancreas, GI, Breast, Bladder, Liver, Leukemia and particularly the Prostate. Doctors in Germany conducted a study examining the relationships between dietary intake of vitamin K1 and K2 on the development of prostate cancer in 11,319 men over an 8.6-year follow-up. Compared with the lowest intake of vitamin K2, men with the highest vitamin K2 dietary consumption showed a 63% reduced incidence of advanced prostate cancer. Intake of vitamin K1 was not related to prostate cancer incidence in this 2008 study. Apatone® is a drug consisting of vitamin C and vitamin K3. It has been granted orphan drug status by the FDA to treat advanced bladder cancer

Vitamin K is actually a group that includes two natural "vitamers", vitamin K_1 and vitamin K_2. Vitamin K_1 is phylloquinone or phytomenadione (also called phytonadione). K_1 is synthesized by plants and is found in green leafy vegetables and can be found in soybean oil. Vitamin K_2 homologs (menaquinones) are characterized by the number of isoprene side chains. These are produced in the intestine from the plant derived K_1 These menaquinones are abbreviated MK-n,(n represents the number of the side chains). Thus, Menaquinone (Vitamin)K-4 abbreviated MK-4, has 4 side chains. Three synthetic types of vitamin K have been made and patented. These are vitamins K_3, K_4, and K_5. Although the natural K_1 and K_2 forms are safe, the synthetic form K_3 (menadione) has shown toxicity. Vitamin K2 shows numerous advantages over vitamin K1, including better absorption, longer lasting and increased protection against heart disease The MK-4 and MK-7 forms of vitamin K2 have demonstrated important health benefits in numerous studies. While the MK-4 form has been shown to support cardiovascular and bone health, the MK-7 form is exceptionally long acting and reaches higher levels in the blood. Therefore when taking a Vitamin K supplement, not only the dose, but the specific subtype is very important.

- Individuals who use Coumadin® have long been advised to avoid vitamin K, and as a result, they may suffer increased atherosclerosis and osteoporosis. Under a doctor's supervision, vitamin K can help stabilize blood indicators of coagulation in Coumadin® users while conferring other health benefits.
- By preventing pathological tissue calcification, vitamin K may confer anti-aging effects throughout the body. Higher vitamin K intake has also been associated with reduced all-cause mortality.

Daily supplementation with vitamin K1 and K2 (in both the MK-4 and MK-7 forms) is crucial for vascular health, bone health, and cancer protection.

Vitamin K2 has proven to be as effective as prescription drugs in reducing the incidence of bone fractures. A Japanese study in postmenopausal women compared the effect of K2 (MK-4) with the drug etidronate (Didronel®) on the incidence of vertebral (spine) fracture. Women taking K2 at a dose of 45 mg per day experienced a fracture rate of 8.0% compared with 8.7% for those taking the etidronate drug therapy. Furthermore, women taking both MK-4 and the drug experienced only a 3.8% fracture rate. In a placebo group that received neither K2 nor drug therapy, nearly 21% of women experienced bone fractures.

FOLIC ACID (FOLACIN OR VITAMIN M)

Folic acid is a coenzyme needed for formation of protein

and hemoglobin. It is available from green vegetables, wheat grains, and brewer's yeast. The best natural source is a fresh green garden salad. Unlike the other water soluble vitamins, folic acid can be stored in the liver so you do not need to eat it every day. It is considered a B vitamin and acts like its cousins, B6 and B12, because a deficiency figures into the homosysteine that causes premature atherosclerosis. Some folks have a genetic problem in converting folic acid to its active form and must take the MethylTetraHydroFolic (MTHF) form. It is available in brands such as Cerafolin.

If a woman doesn't have enough of it during early pregnancy, neural tube defects in the baby are the result. In doses of 5 mg a day, it is used to treat otherwise refractory arthritis and pain problems. It promotes healthy skin and improves the appetite in cases of debilitation. The FDA recently increased the RDA from 200 to 400 mg daily, and since 1998 it has been used to fortify cereals and grain products. Studies show that women who are at risk of pregnancy should take extra folic acid rather than wait until after their pregnancy is suspected or confirmed. Study after study shows that extra folic acid prevents cancer.

Biotin

Biotin is used in the body for synthesis of ascorbic acid. The best natural sources are nuts, fruits, brewer's yeast, and unpolished rice. It is essential for the normal metabolism of fats and proteins. It maintains healthy skin and is especially good for the health of hair follicles. This vitamin will rejuvenate hair follicles when taken by mouth or rubbed directly on the skin in a cream base. It may even regrow a few hairs that have gone into early retirement. Hair will stand up straighter and have a healthier sheen. It is given in doses of 200 to 2000 mcg per day. It is also good for nails.

CHOLINE

Choline is found in lecithin, brewer's yeast, fish tofu, tempeh, miso, peanuts, beef liver, egg yolk, wheat germ, cauliflower, and cabbage. This B type vitamin is an antioxidant and a membrane stabilizer. It is used for transport and metabolism of fats and cholesterol in the liver. It may prevent cardiovascular disease, and it detoxifies the liver and facilitates transmission of nerve impulses. It prevents and treats memory loss and diseases of the nervous system, and can influence mood and depression, as well as strengthen capillary walls and accelerate blood flow, thereby lowering blood pressure. Also, it has been used in the treatment of gallstones.

Deficiency symptoms are high blood pressure, bleeding ulcers, coronary artery disease, hemorrhaging of the kidneys, atherosclerosis, headaches, dizziness, ear noises, palpitations, and constipation. Choline seems to work better when taken with biotin. It is used as an aid to weight loss.

VITAMIN CoQ10 (UBIQUINOL)

The late Dr. Carl Fokers, considered the Linus Pauling of CoQ10, repeatedly requested that this substance be elevated to the status of a vitamin. There have been solid scientific studies on the mechanism and actions of CoQ10 since the early 1970s. The body makes some CoQ10 for basic functioning but not enough during times of mental and physical stress. It acts as a premiere antioxidant and has no negative side effects—but it is expensive.

An Italian study of 2,664 patients with heart failure—hearts that weren't pumping strong enough to keep up with bodily demands—showed that those given an average of 100 mg had a marked improvement compared with patients not taking it. Langsjoen published a positive study on coenzyme CoQ10 for treatment of dilated cardiomyopathy, which is a heart unable to pump well enough to keep up with the needs of the body.

Interest in this chemical was stimulated by the discovery, in 1961, that blood levels of CoQ10 correlate with cancer and the stage of the cancer. Breast cancer, for instance, is associated with a decrease in the blood level of CoQ10. In cancers with a bad prognosis, there is a dramatic decrease in CoQ10 levels. CoQ10 can slow progression of cancer and its use as an alternative or adjunct to radiation and chemotherapy is warranted. It stimulates the immune system and aids the body to heal itself. The dose is 60 mg to 300 mg a day.

Bioflavonoids (Vitamin P)

The bioflavonoids (flavonoids, isoflavones) are polyphenolic antioxidants found in fruits and vegetables. Major sources are tea, onions, apples, yams, cucumbers, citrus fruits, and berries. Although there are various types such as kaempferol, myricetin, apigenin, luteolin, proanthycyanidin, the most popular is quercetin. Proanthycanidin is distributed in the United States under the name Adoxynol. Dr. David White, a researcher at the University of Nottingham in England, says Vitamin P is fifty times more powerful than Vitamin E.

Without flavonoids, some say, vitamin C is mostly oxidized and less useful. The flavonoids protect the integrity of the capillary wall, reduce blood clots, and inhibit plaque formation in arteries. It also reduces the body's ability to absorb cholesterol from food, according to Dr. T. Chisaka at the Kyoto Pharmaceutical University in Japan.

Dr. Michael Herzog headed a study of more than 12,000 elderly men conducted by the public health divisions of seven European countries. The study showed that a high intake of flavonoids resulted in a 50 percent less risk of having heart problems compared to those with a low intake.

In a study published in *Lancet* of 805 males aged fifty-five to sixty-four, there was an inverse relationship between the amount of flavonoids ingested over the previous five years by a cross-check dietary history and coronary artery disease. In addition, flavonoids have been shown to be anti-inflammatory and they decrease the incidence of viral infections.

PABA (PARA-AMINO BUTYRIC ACID)

PABA is found in liver, brewer's yeast, wheat germ, molasses, eggs, organ meats, yogurt, and green leafy vegetables. PABA stimulates intestinal bacteria, which aids in production of pantothenic acid. It is a coenzyme in making blood cells and metabolizing protein and is important for skin health, hair pigmentation, and the health of the intestines. It may also help with vitiligo, restore hair from graying, and is used for many skin conditions. It protects against ozone toxicity.

PABA deficiency causes symptoms similar to those of folic acid or pantothenic acid deficiency; it also causes vitiligo, fatigue, irritability, depression, nervousness, headache, constipation, and other digestive disorders.

VITAMIN T

Known as the "sesame seed factor," Vitamin T is found in sesame seeds and egg yolks. We do not yet know exactly what this substance is, but it is thought to be helpful in preventing anemia and the destruction of red blood cells. Halava, a high-protein food made from sesame seeds, helped keep the armies marching in the time of Alexander the Great.

VITAMIN U

As with Vitamin T, not much is known about Vitamin U. It is found in raw cabbage, has no known toxicity, and may be helpful in healing ulcers of the skin and intestinal tract. The active nutrient is probably allantoin, which has tissue-healing power. It is also found in herbs such as comfrey root, which is known to help heal and soothe the gastrointestinal mucosa. Cabbage, commonly consumed in long-living groups such as the Hunzas, is thought to be a very important enzyme food.

Multivitamin Pills and Capsules

It is impossible to get all your necessary vitamins and dietary supplements in one pill. There are products on the market that try to supply everything in three to fifteen pills a day. To make supplement taking easier, several products are placed in several capsules, some liquid/gel, others powder/granule-filled. To help make you more accountable and keep it convenient, three or four pills and capsules are usually placed in clear packets to be taken at several appropriate times a day. Another method is to place the powder and liquid products in a drink with macronutrient liquids such as whey or low carbohydrate fluid and mix with some ice to make a smoothie. To be very frugal, twice a day Centrum Silver (or similar) vitamins might suffice. Being a synthetic product or "non-dissolvable" makes little difference because much of the active material is leached out of the capsule by the body.

Minerals

Boron

Found in fresh fruits and vegetables, boron helps retain calcium in bones, prevents calcium and magnesium loss through the urine, helps bone mineralization, and prevents osteoporosis. In post-menopausal women, it increases estrogen naturally. Deficiency symptoms have not been officially recognized. The optimal daily amount is 1 to 3 mg, combined with calcium and magnesium. No RDA has been established.

Calcium

Calcium is found in milk, egg yolk, fish or sardines (eaten with bones), yogurt, soybeans, green leafy vegetables such as turnip greens, mustard greens, broccoli and kale, roots, tubers, seeds, soups and stews made from bones, blackstrap molasses, almonds, figs, and beans. Recent literature suggests calcium from milk sources may actually cause osteoporosis. Calcium maintains acid-alkaline balance in the body and normalizes contraction and relaxation of the heart and skeletal muscles. It strengthens bones and teeth, therefore protecting against osteoporosis, rickets, and osteomalacia (bone-softening disease). It lowers high blood pressure and cholesterol and aids in preventing cardiovascular disease. With vitamin C, it relieves backaches, menstrual cramps, and sleep problems. It may help prevent colorectal cancer.

The deficiency symptoms are nervous spasms, facial twitching, weak muscles, cramps, rickets and slow growth in children, osteoporosis, osteomalacia, palpitations and slow pulse rate, height reduction, and colon cancer.

The optimal daily amount is 1,000 to 1,500 mg with equal parts of magnesium. Some researchers say menopausal women need 1,500 mg, with added boron and magnesium. RDA is 1,000 mg daily for adults, 1,200 mg during pregnancy and lactation, and 1,200 mg for ages eleven to twenty-four.

CHLORIDE

Since chloride is found in salt (sodium chloride) and salt substitutes (potassium chloride), we seldom need supplementation. Chloride stimulates production of hydrochloric acid for digestion and maintains fluid and electrolyte balance. Chloride has also been shown to assist liver function.

The deficiency symptoms, although rare as the body usually produces enough, include impaired digestion and loss of hair and teeth. The optimal daily amount has not been established. Do not confuse chloride with chlorine, an active form of chloride used in American water purification systems, which is indeed dangerous.

CHROMIUM

Found in brewer's yeast, blackstrap molasses, black pepper, meat (especially liver), whole wheat bread and cereals, beets, and mushrooms. Chromium helps stabilize blood sugar levels, therefore being effective against diabetes and hypoglycemia. It aids in lowering cholesterol and increases the level of high-density lipoproteins (HDLs) in humans (shown to be protective against cardiovascular disease). Chromium can increase lean muscle tissue while decreasing body fat. Deficiency symptoms include slowed growth, shortened lifespan, raised cholesterol levels, and an array of symptoms related to low and high blood sugar such as diabetes. The optimal daily amount is 200 to 400 mcg. Chromium polynicotinate, which is considered better than chromium picolinate, are both natural forms. The RDA has not been established. The National Research Council tentatively recommends 500 to 2,300 mcg daily for diabetics.

COPPER

Copper is found in nuts, organ meats, seafood, mushrooms, and legumes. Accompanied by iron and protein, it aids in synthesizing red blood cells. It forms melanin (pigment in skin and hair) and helps to make connective tissues such as collagen and elastin. Copper assists in lowering cholesterol, improves the immune system, and maintains cellular structure. It may help as an anti-inflammatory for arthritics, particularly if used topically (such as in bracelets).

Deficiency symptoms include neuropathy, mild anemia, loss of hair, loss of taste, general weakness, impaired respiration, brittle bones, chronic or recurrent diarrhea, premature graying of hair, low white blood cell count, retarded growth, water retention, irritability, high cholesterol, abnormal EGG patterns, ischemic heart disease, birth defects, miscarriage, and neural tube defects. Antacid use creates copper deficiency. Very high amounts of copper can cause mood swings and depression, in addition to insomnia, painful joints, and mental and physical fatigue. Extra exposure to copper comes from cookware, hair sprays, deodorants, and copper water pipes. The optimal daily amount is 2 to 3 mg taken with zinc at a 10:1 or 15:1 zinc to copper ratio. RDA is 2 mg.

Fluoride

Often added to municipal drinking water, fluoride is thought to be necessary for the formation of strong bones and teeth and may protect against osteoporosis. Too much, however, may cause fatigue, muscle pain, mottled teeth, and even cancer. There are no deficiency states and hence no optimal daily amount. Do not take additional fluoride. It is found in various toothpastes and mouthwashes. Because of problems with excess fluoride producing the above symptoms (fluoridosis), many health care workers lobby against adding it to drinking water. In high doses, for which a prescription is needed, it has been used to improve bone mineral density, but today we know that it only makes bones *appear* better on X-rays. They are still just as weak.

Germanium

Germanium is a trace mineral occurring naturally in very small amounts in the soil and in certain foods and herbs, such as shiitake mushrooms, ginseng root, garlic, shelf fungus, and aloe vera. It has been used for its semiconductor properties in making computer chips. In humans, the organic form has a variety of health-giving effects. Germanium has immunological functions, such as stimulating interferon, as well as macrophage and natural killer lymphocyte activity. There is some suggestion that germanium helps in pain relief; particularly dramatic relief has occurred in some cases of severe cancer pain. It is also part of the cancer cure cocktail. In both sick and normal humans, Germanium is virtually nontoxic. Germanium is currently considered a food supplement and is available in health food stores. Make sure that it is in the organo-germanium sesquioxide form. Amounts in supplements range from 25 to 150 mg; up to 1 to 6 grams daily may be needed for pain or cancer. Allergies have also been reduced by the use of this nutrient, particularly those allergies arising from foods.

Hydrochloric Acid (HCl)

As mentioned earlier in the book, hydrochloric acid is greatly reduced in 30 percent of individuals older than sixty years of age. Decreased HCl production leads to poor digestion, with symptoms such as gas, bloating, and discomfort after rich meals. Some symptoms may actually mimic an ulcer, and folks erroneously take ulcer medicine, supressing the acid even more. An HCl supplement may improve digestion of meals containing protein and/or fat, though not for foods such as rice and vegetables, which are largely carbohydrates and thus need less HCl for digestion.

Hydrochloric acid is available primarily as betaine hydrochloride. When a 5 to 10 grain (1 grain = 64 mg) tablet is taken during a meal, it should help proteins break down into peptide sand amino acids and fats into triglycerides. I ask my patients to increase the number of pills, even up to five at a time, if a lower number of pills do not work. Low HCl production is associated with many problems, including iron deficiency anemia, B12 deficiency, osteoporosis, and fatigue. With low stomach acid levels, there is an increase of bacteria, yeasts, and parasites growing in the intestines. HCl is a stimulus to pancreatic secretions that contain the majority of enzymes that actively breaks down foods. Without HCl, the whole digestive system performs poorly. It is the key that unlocks the door to digestion.

IRON

Iron is found in many foods, including liver, heart, kidney, lean meats, shellfish, dried beans, fruit, nuts, leafy vegetables, whole grains, and blackstrap molasses. Iron is the essential mineral in hemoglobin and the red pigment in muscles. It can cure and prevent iron-deficiency anemia and stimulates immunity. Iron is needed in muscular and athletic performance and is an aid in preventing fatigue.

Symptoms of deficiency include anemia (pallor, weakness, persistent fatigue, labored breathing on exertion, headaches, and palpitation). Young children suffer diminished coordination, as well as decrease attention span and memory; older children have poor learning, reading, and problem-solving skills; depressed immune system with decreased ability to produce white blood cells for fighting off infection; concave or spoonlike fingernails and toenails. The optimal daily amount (RDA) is 10 mg for men and 18 mg for women. As a supplement, *do not use* inorganic iron (ferrous sulfate) with vitamin E. Use, instead, the organic iron compounds ferrous fumarate, ferrous citrate, or ferrous gluconate. Men and non-menstruating women should not take extra iron products because it causes premature atherosclerosis since it is an oxidant. Individuals with low iron are pale (Plummer-Vincent Syndrome) have fingernail concavity and esophageal webs, which make swallowing difficult. As noted later in this book, some people who appear to have iron deficiency anemia do not respond until molybdenum is added to the regimen.

LITHIUM

This metal is found in small amounts in fish, processed meats, dairy products, eggs, potatoes, and some vegetables. Even with eating these foods, you will receive less than one-tenth of what is needed to keep your brain working the best it can. Over two thousand years ago, it was noticed that the waters of certain mineral springs seemed to have curative powers for people suffering from "nerves." In the second century AD, the Greek physician Seranus Ephesios recommended "natural waters such as alkaline springs" as a treatment for mania. Over the ensuing two millennia, countless people have "taken the waters" for a variety of ailments, real and imagined, at fashionable (and not so fashionable) spas throughout the world, particularly in Europe. Lithium is so effective in controlling the mood extremes of bipolar disorder that to this day it is still used in the treatment of both manic and manic-depressive disease. The fact that lithium controls both mania and depression (the former more effectively than the latter) is both wonderful and puzzling, as it suggests that both of these conditions are, somehow, symptoms of the same underlying neurochemical disturbance.

Lithium's mechanism of action on the brain is still unknown and speculative; it may affect the levels of the neurotransmitters serotonin and norepinephrine in the brain. There is also evidence that lithium inhibits the action of inositol monophosphatase and several other enzymes that play key roles in mood-related neuromodulation (a complex type of signaling process related to neurotransmission). Also in Alzheimer's, there is a decrease of the amyloid/beta plaques and neuro-fibrillatory tangles that are the hallmark of this disorder. Lithium protects against neuronal death, very much like the drug for Alzheimer's disease, Namenda, by decreasing glutamate-induced exitotoxicity. The latter is caused by our neurotransmitters because of stress and is a cause of Alzheimer's. Excessive amounts of glutamate, the brain's most prevalent transmitter, damages our brain cells. Lithium stimulates the protective brain-derived neurotropic factor (BDNF), which is essential for the development and maintenance of healthy neurons. BDNF also helps increase white blood cells.

One further mechanism has been described recently. Lithium stimulates the growth of new brain cells, a process called neurogenesis. It increases the grey matter, which is mostly the supporting tissue, the glial cells, we now feel play a role in the maintenance of a healthy brain. This drug/supplement was in the past thought to be helpful in the preservation of the neurons in multiple sclerosis and ALS, but recent double-blind studies showed little or no effect.

Medically, only lithium carbonate in therapeutic doses are used. This requires a prescription. It is very inexpensive in that it has been generic for the last twenty-five years. The dose of 600 to 1,200 mg daily is usually required for the treatment of mania.

It is important that the blood is monitored periodically so that the therapeutic range of .5 to 1.5 mm/l is obtained. If lower than this, there may be poor results. If higher, there may be negative effects on the kidneys and tremors and psychosis may result. Even in the desired range, after many months lithium can cause low thyroid, and this, too, must be monitored. Much smaller doses of other nonprescriptive lithium salts such as orate, aspartate, and chloride are used with varying success. I have used 300 to 350 mg daily of the prescription without monitoring. Time will tell if this will help those who ask for it, but at least it is safe and inexpensive.

MAGNESIUM

In a recent study, 75 percent of Americans were found to be deficient in magnesium because our soil has been depleted of this important mineral. Drugs such as diuretics, cortisone, and aminophylline also lower our body's magnesium content. Magnesium improves one's insulin and cholesterol metabolism and hence, will lower blood sugar and cholesterol. It is now thought to be as important as calcium in preventing osteoporosis. It has also been used successfully to treat PMS, mitral valve prolapse, kidney stones, hypertension, and migraine headaches. Deficiency syndromes include heart problems, apathy, depression, kidney stones, disorientation, muscle weakness and spasms, poor memory, irritability, tremors, and even seizures. Magnesium functions as a catalyst in over 1,000 of our enzyme systems.

Although magnesium can be found in foods including chard, pinto beans, avocados, and oatmeal, I recommend supplements. There are many products on the market such as Slo-Mag, Mag-L, K-Mag, Magna Magtab SR, and my favorite, Mag Citrate. These can be purchased in health food stores or inexpensively from the hardware store in the form of epsom salts (magnesium sulfate) and a teaspoon, two or three times a day, can supply you with the correct amount of magnesium. However, people occasionally do get a little diarrhea with this. Periodically, the clinician should do a magnesium level to make sure the level is good without excess. However, in general, magnesium is a very safe mineral. I recommend the white blood cell magnesium test, as this reflects the true body amount. The RDA is 400 mg daily, and our diet supplies only half of that. Taken before bedtime gives a better night's sleep.

Manganese

Manganese is found in whole grains, peas, nuts, leafy green vegetables, egg yolk, bananas, organ meats, and milk. It is required for vital enzyme reaction and proper bone development as well as synthesis of mucopoly saccharides. It is helpful in preventing osteoarthritis and is required for many enzyme reactions. The normal functioning of the pancreas needs manganese, as does carbohydrate metabolism. It plays an important part in the formation of thyroxin, a hormone secreted by the thyroid gland. It may also improve memory and reduce nervous irritability. Calm (magnesium citrate) can help mitigate the effects of migraine headaches.

Deficiency symptoms include weight loss, dermatitis, nausea, slow growth, and color changes of hair, low cholesterol, as well as disturbances in fat metabolism and glucose tolerance. Deficiency is suspected in diabetes, and deficiency during pregnancy may be a factor in epilepsy in the offspring. Too much manganese can cause hypertension and irreversible movement disorders. Optimal daily amount is 5 to 10 mg in combination with other minerals. No RDA has been established.

Molybdenum

Molybdenum is found in organ meats, dairy products, legumes, whole grains, and leafy green vegetables. This mineral is required for the activity of several enzymes in the body, including the enzyme responsible for iron utilization. It helps not only to prevent anemia, but treats refractory patients that are misdiagnosed as having iron deficiency. Molybdenum detoxifies potentially hazardous substances with which one may come in contact. It can be an antioxidant and protects teeth from cavities. It also aids in carbohydrate and fat metabolism.

Deficiency symptoms include possible esophageal cancer in those who eat plants from molybdenum-deficient soil. Optimal intake is still uncertain, but 50 to 200 mcg (not mg) is suggested. No RDA has been established.

Phosphorous

Phosphorous is found in high-protein foods such as meat, fish, poultry, eggs, milk, cheese, nuts, legumes, and bone meal. Many processed foods and soft drinks preserved with phosphates adversely affect the body's calcium-phosphorous balance. Phosphorous is essential for bone mineralization and tooth structure. It may reduce muscular fatigue and is involved in cellular activity. It has been shown to be important for heart regularity and needed for the transference of nerve impulses. It also aids in growth and body repair.

Deficiency symptoms include muscle weakness to the point of respiratory arrest, anemia, increased susceptibility to infections, and hemorrhage. The typical American diet makes a phosphorous deficiency rare in the United States, although those with kidney failure or those who drink large quantities of soft drinks can have too much. Diabetics, alcoholics, persons with diarrheal diseases, and those taking antacids may be deficient. No supplementation is generally needed, as the diet should supply sufficient amounts. RDA is 800 to 1,200 mg for adults.

Potassium

Potassium is found in bananas, apricots, lettuce, broccoli, potatoes, fresh fruits and fruit juices, sunflower seeds, unsalted peanuts, nuts, squash, wheat germ, brewers yeast, liver, fish, bone meal, watercress, blackstrap molasses, and tea. Potassium helps balance fluid with sodium inside the cells, and it is used by the body for proper muscle and heart contraction. It helps red blood cells in carrying oxygen and eliminating water waste through the kidneys. It is used in carbohydrate metabolism and energy storage in the muscles and liver. It reduces high blood pressure, allergies, and colic in babies, and it is important for those using diuretics. Finally, it keeps the heart in rhythm.

Deficiency symptoms include general weakness of muscles, mental confusion, muscle cramping, poor reflexes, nervous system disruption, soft, flabby muscles, constipation, and acne in young people and dry skin in adults. Severe deficiency or excess leads to cardiac arrest. The optimal daily amount is 2,000 to 4,000 mg. Generally one gets enough from foods. Athletes, however, generally require more (3,000 to 6,000 mg) because of heavy perspiration. The maximum potency allowed by the government in supplement form is 99 mg. An inexpensive and effective replacement is the product *Nu-Salt* or *No-Salt* obtained in the grocery store rather than the health food or drugstore.

Discuss higher potencies with a physician. RDA is 2,000 to 2,500 mg. Expect the doctor to talk in milliequivalents (meq).

SELENIUM

This is found in organ meats, tuna, seafood, brewer's yeast, fresh garlic, mushrooms, wheat germ, and some whole grains. Selenium is necessary for the body's growth and protein synthesis. It helps to increase effectiveness of vitamin E. An antioxidant for the cells to protect against oxygen exposure, it also protects against toxic pollutants (especially mercury) for sexual reproduction. Selenium may reduce risk of cancer and help against abnormal heart rhythm. It has been shown to alleviate hot flashes and some menopausal symptoms, as well as reduce free-radical damage that causes aging. It neutralizes heavy metal toxcities such as mercury and lead. *Selenomethionine* is an amino acid containing selentium that is much better absorbed and more effective than other selenium products.

Deficiency symptoms include dandruff, ozone damage to the lungs, decreased growth, infant deaths associated with selenium and/or vitamin E deficiency, and increased risk of cancer and heart disease. The optimal daily amount is 100 to 200 ug in high selenium areas and 200 to 400 ug in low selenium areas. The Food and Nutrition Board states that overt selenium toxicity may occur in humans ingesting 3,000 ug a day. No RDA has been established. Up to 2 grams a day have been used in a series of cancer patients without apparent toxicity. For many years I have prescribed 600 ug of selenium for patients with disordered heart rhythm.

SILVER

Silver has been used since antiquity for its healing and preserving powers. The ancient Greeks kept their medicinal liquids (and expensive foods) free of contamination by placing them in silver jars. Since the Middle Ages, silver was a staple for cookware and people usually ate with silver pans, plates, and utensils. Silver and its salts have been used for centuries for disease treatment; 150 years ago for syphilis; in the last hundred years for eye and nose drops, gargles, and douches; and in the most recent forty years topically for burns and skin ulcers. It is also now used as the material from which medical devices are made, including urinary and venous catheters as well as surgical instruments by mainstream physicians.

Silver and its compounds have electrical/oligodynamic effects that are toxic for bacteria, algae, fungi, and some parasites. This is typical for heavy metals like lead and mercury. Among the elements that have this, silver is the least toxic for humans. The medicinal action of silver is dependent on the electrical aspects of the silver ion, which irreversibly damages key enzyme systems in the cell membrane of certain pathogens to include staph and the internal organization of some viruses.

Today colloidal silver is made in ultramicroscopic particles in a solution suspended naturally in deionized water by natural electromagnetic charges. This ultra-fine 99.999 percent silver has a particle size from 0.0001 to 0.001 microns (1 to 100 ug). A red blood cell is a giant compared to this, being 7 microns or seven million times bigger! After ingestion, this metal enters the bloodstream within twenty minutes and is dispersed all over the body. Colloidal silver can be obtained for less than $4 an ounce at health food stores. Or with equipment costing less than $100, one can make gallons of it for $5. Since it is light-sensitive, silver should be kept in darkly tinted glass bottles in a cool place. Plastic containers magnetize easily and the silver particles will stick to the sides. Also keep it away from magnetic fields such as electronics or motors since they will interfere with the ions, holding the colloid in solution. If placed in the refrigerator, the silver may fall out of solution.

Colloidal silver is predictably safe. As a pre-1938 medicinal, it is out of the control of the FDA. In general, silver exhibits low toxicity in the human body, and minimal risk is expected due to excess intake. Argyria is usually benign and limited to blue skin discoloration. There are isolated reports of more serious neurologic (seizures), renal, or hepatic complications, as well as headaches, stomach distress, fatigue, and skin irritation. Colloidal silver may react with certain drugs, such as thyroid and antibiotics (quinalones and tetracyclines). The reference dose, published by the EPA (the daily exposure that is unlikely to incur a appreciable risk of deleterious effects during a lifetime) is 5 μg/kg daily; meaning 5 micrograms of silver per kilo of weight per person each day—about 1 liter of 10 ppm colloidal silver per month for a 66 kg person.

In order to guarantee the effectiveness of colloidal silver, it is necessary to buy a product that provides ten particles of silver per million of water. Do not consume more than a quart daily for safety's sake. Review the label or the specifications in the literature with the product. It is essential to get this health supplement from suppliers that have good feedback from customers and the above specifications. Some suppliers, like American Biotech Labs, combine oxygen with purified silver, which is said to disrupt the pathogen's ability to produce energy even more and increases the bioavailability of the silver particles.

My opinion on colloidal silver is not as bullish as it was a decade ago. There has never been a good randomized double-blind study to support it in evidence-based medicine, but in my experience (experience-based medicine), it should be considered in mild infections when antibiotics are not only more expensive but more dangerous! It should also be considered in hard-to-eradicate infections, along with other maladies such as HIV and Lyme disease. No doubt it is very helpful when used topically in wounds. Again, watch the label for 10 ppm and 5 ng particle size, and no more than a quart a day! My colleagues may not agree with me, but for those who *believe*, no evidence is necessary. For those who do *not* believe, no evidence is sufficient.

Silicon (Silica)

This is found in horsetail (an herb), flaxseed, steel cut oats, almonds, peanuts, sunflower seeds, onions, alfalfa, fresh fruit, brewer's yeast, and dietary fiber. Silicon can help build connective tissue and helps with hair, skin, and nails.

Deficiency symptoms are aging of skin (wrinkles), thinning or loss of hair, poor bone development, and soft or brittle nails. No dietary recommendations are given for this mineral. Adequate amounts are found in the diet, therefore no RDA has been established.

Sodium

Sodium is found in sea salt, shellfish, meat, poultry, milk, cheese, kelp, powdered seaweed, and most processed foods. Sodium works with potassium to maintain proper fluid balance between cells. It is also used for nerve stimulation for muscle contraction and helps in keeping calcium and other minerals soluble in the blood. Sodium stimulates the adrenal glands and helps strengthen weak muscles. High sodium may account for high blood pressure and osteoporosis. Finally, sodium aids in preventing heat prostration or sunstroke.

Deficiency is rare since most foods contain sodium, however, symptoms include headaches, excessive sweating, heat exhaustion, respiratory failure, muscular cramps, weakness, collapsed blood vessels, stomach and intestinal gas, chronic diarrhea, weight loss, kidney failure, and a tendency for infections. RDA is 200 to 600 mg. In our modern society, we take too much of this mineral into our bodies. Home water softeners, prepared foods, and our own salt shakers are the worst offenders. If we did not have any salt consumption, there would be no hypertension, say some experts.

Sulfur

Sulphur is found in protein foods, especially egg yolks, lean beef, fish, onions, kale, soybeans, and dried beans. Sulfur is in every cell of the body, helping the nerves and muscles function properly and normalizing glandular secretions. It is necessary for healthy hair, skin, and nails. It also helps maintain oxygen balance necessary for brain function. The homeopathic remedy of sulfur helps with rashes, itching and other skin conditions. Deficiency symptoms are rare but may be excessive sweating, chronic diarrhea, nausea, respiratory failure, heat exhaustion, muscular weakness, and mental apathy. A diet sufficient in protein should be adequate in sulfur. No RDA has been established. MSM is an excellent source of sulfur.

Vanadium

The richest sources of vanadium are fish, black pepper, and dill seed, middle range includes whole grains, meats, and dairy products. Research shows that vanadium improves glucose tolerance and improves insulin efficiency in diabetics. Deficiency symptoms are little known at this time, but high blood pressure and hardening of the arteries have been suggested. No RDA has been established, but 10 to 50 mg a day of vanadium sulfate is recommended for diabetics.

Zinc

Zinc is found in fresh oysters (which could be dangerous to eat), herring, wheat germ, pumpkin seeds, milk, steamed crab, lobster, chicken, pork chops, turkey and ground beef, liver, and eggs. Zinc helps promote wound healing and improves various skin disorders, including acne. It affects impotence in men by increasing sperm count. It helps with prostate enlargement. It may be used for combating colds and flu to increase immunity. It may help with some forms of cancer and, with antioxidants, it retards macular degeneration.

Deficiency symptoms are fingernails with white spots or bands and an opaquely white appearance, loss of taste, smell, and appetite, delayed sexual development in adolescence, underdeveloped penis, and less full beard and underarm hair in boys, irregular menstrual cycle in girls, infertility and impaired sexual function in adults, poor wound healing. loss of hair, increased susceptibility to infection, reduced salivation, skin lesions; stretch marks, reduced absorption of nutrients, impaired development of bones, muscles, and nervous system, deformed offspring, and dwarfism. Given to a teenager, it might make the youngster taller. Normal daily amount is 30 to 50 mg (take with copper, a zinc:copper ratio of 10:1). RDA is 15 mg. I frequently prescribe zinc for short time periods, 200 to 250 mg a day.

NOTES

1   A stool study for less than $100 can be ordered online from www.
    enterolab.com, or your doctor can contact the Intestinal Health
    Institute, P.O. Box 570744, Dallas, TX, 75357. This test is called an
    antigliadin antibody test. It is only positive if the individual is still
    eating gluten. From the stool, genetic studies can also be done for
    another $50 even if the patient is gluten-free. Ninety eight percent
    of patients who have celiac disease have HLA-DQ2 or HLA-DQ8
    haplotype.
        An even better test is the Celiac Plus® from Prometheus (888-
    423-0896 or 888-423-0896), which does all the antibodies and
    the genetic haplotype test. It will also identify the more aggressive
    disease variant by identifying the dreaded DQB1*0201 gene.
    Costing $500, it might be the best money spent to pin down this
    disease, possibly preventing disability and even death, secondary
    to cancer! Also, many insurance plans pay for it.

2   *Archives of Internal Medicine*, September 25, 2000, 260:2641–44.

3   *Neurology*, 52:1563–69.

4   *American Journal of Nutrition*, 2000, 71(2):480–84.

5   *Archives of Ophthalmology*, 2000, 118:1556–63.

6   A former student of mine, Gino Tuttera, MD, has personally
    implanted more than ten thousand of these without event. His
    website for more information is SottoPelle.com.

7   Diane Feskanich, *American Journal of Epidemiology*, 143:5.

8   *The Journal of Science*, January 16, 1998.

9   Dr. P. J. Tutbaugh, *Nature*, December 21, 2006.

INDEX